Geographic Medicine for the Practitioner

Studies in Infectious Disease Research

Edward H. Kass, M.D., General Editor

Geographic Medicine for the Practitioner

Algorithms in the

Diagnosis and Management of Exotic Diseases

Edited by Kenneth S. Warren and Adel A. F. Mahmoud

The University of Chicago Press

Chicago and London

1978

The material presented in this volume was originally published
serially in the *Journal of Infectious Diseases,* Volume 132, number
5 through volume 136, number 4.

The University of Chicago Press, Chicago 60637
The University of Chicago Press, Ltd., London

Library of Congress Cataloging in Publication Data
Main entry under title:

Geographic medicine and the practitioner.

  Revised version of articles first published in
the Journal of infectious diseases 1975-1977.
  Includes bibliographical references and index.
  1. Communicable diseases—Addresses, essays,
lectures.   2. Tropical medicine—Addresses, essays,
lectures.   3. Travel—Hygienic aspects—Addresses,
essays, lectures.   I. Warren, Kenneth S.
II. Mahmoud, Adel A. F.   III. Title: Exotic diseases.
[DNLM: 1. Communicable diseases—Collected works.
WC100 W289g]
RC111.G46   619.9'88   77-17007
ISBN 0-226-87386-2

Contents

Foreword

The many diseases that are endemic in most of the developing nations of the world (and that may also affect travelers to these regions) are, at world levels, the most important sources of morbidity that affect the entire human race. The change in morbidity patterns in the more developed nations should not be permitted to blind the more affluent countries to the implications of this simple statement. Thus, direct and useful guides are needed to assure efficient and economical diagnosis and treatment of those infections that are endemic to the less affluent two-thirds of the earth.

The algorithms in this book have been developed by Drs. Warren and Mahmoud, as the result of a systematic effort to produce such guides. The book is presented as another in the series "Studies in Infectious Disease Research" and is a most welcome addition, certain to supply a major and hitherto inadequately fulfilled need.

Edward H. Kass, M.D., Ph.D.
General Editor

Preface

The Division of Geographic Medicine at Case Western Reserve University School of Medicine began a cooperative venture in 1975 to prepare a series of succinct articles on exotic viral, bacterial, protozoan, and helminthic infections for publication in the Journal of Infectious Diseases. These infections were considered to be exotic for two reasons: they either came from foreign shores or they were foreign to the information base of the average practitioner.

With respect to an exotic origin for these infections, perusal of U.S. government statistics was startling to say the least—American citizens traveling to areas where these diseases abound (usually the tropics) have averaged approximately 4.5 million trips annually for the last 3 years for a total of over 13 million. Over a similar 3-year period of time, travelers to the United States from endemic areas have included 1 million legal immigrants and 6 million transient visitors. [1] The single most dangerous of these infections is malaria, which is now averaging about 500 cases yearly in the United States; it is important to realize that infection with one species of this organism (*Plasmodium falciparum*) can be lethal within a few days of the onset of fever. Highly contagious infections such as smallpox (almost, but not quite eradicated), and the newly discovered, extremely lethal Lassa fever may be imported to our shores, plus cholera, antibiotic-resistant bacillary dysentery, and amebic dysentery and liver abscess. Chronic worm infections such as schistosomiasis, while rarely lethal, may occasion uncomfortable, invasive diagnostic procedures and the use of toxic drugs for their treatment.

It is worthy of note that certain of these so-called "exotic infections" are widely spread throughout the United States or are highly endemic in particular regions. With respect to the former, it has been estimated that pinworms infect 42 million Americans in every state including Alaska, and trichinosis and tapeworms are also distributed widely, but at relatively low levels of prevalence. [2] Toxoplasmosis, an infection that may cause birth defects and blindness,

has infected over 30% of our population; giardiasis is now considered by the Center for Disease Control to be the most common cause of water-borne epidemics of diarrhea in the United States; and *Entamoeba histolytica* infects at least 5% of Americans. [3] In the southwestern states, hookworm, whipworm, and the foot-long intestinal roundworm (*Ascaris*) are prevalent; and in certain southwestern states the highly dangerous hydatid cyst of *Echinococcus granulosus* has now been shown to be endemic. Bubonic plague is spread throughout the rodents of the western states, and some human infections and fatalities are reported annually. Furthermore, it must always be kept in mind that patients immunosuppressed either by certain disease states or by therapy to prevent graft rejection are susceptible to fatal opportunistic infections with certain of these agents (e.g., *Strongyloides* or *Toxoplasma*).

In spite of the vast global prevalence of these infections and the presence of many of them in the United States, a recent survey has revealed that these so-called "tropical diseases" are taught superficially in most American medical schools (1–10 hours of lectures in 56%), and, in 5%, not at all. [4]

When a patient is suspected of suffering from one of the exotic infections, it would be helpful if the physician had a clear, unambiguous source of information on the infection, its disease syndromes and the means of coping with them. When he turns to the usual textbook of tropical medicine or clinical parasitology, however, the practitioner is confronted with a detailed discussion including all of the minutiae of morphology, life cycle, epidemiology, and presumed disease syndromes. When he arrives at methods of diagnosis, he is often referred to an appendix in which multiple procedures are described, each involving equipment and supplies that may not be readily obtainable. Serologic and skin tests are frequently recommended, but the antigens are rarely available. The descriptions of treatment may be even more frustrating, since as many as 10 different drug regimens may be described with no criteria for selection among them, and with frequent mention of drugs that are unlicensed or unavailable.

In an attempt to solve these problems, an abbreviated format has been developed in which the basic facts of life cycle and epidemiology are briefly described and the disease syndromes, diagnosis, and treatment are presented in the form of an algorithm. As described in a recent editorial in the *New England Journal of Medicine,* algorithms should be "unam-

Table 1. Major Areas of Distribution of the Exotic Infections

Worldwide	Africa	Asia	Latin America
Hepatitis	Smallpox	Plague	Yellow fever
Cholera	Yellow fever	Leishmaniasis	Plague*
Leprosy	Lassa fever	Malaria	Leishmaniasis
Shigellosis	Plague	Filariasis	Malaria
Tuberculosis	Leishmaniasis	Clonorchiasis	Trypanosomiasis, Am.
Typhoid	Malaria	Opisthorchiasis	Filariases
Amebiasis	Trypanosomiasis, Afr.	Fasciolopsiasis	Schistosomiasis†
Giardiasis	Filariases	Paragonimiasis	
Toxoplasmosis	Paragonimiasis	Schistosomiasis	
Ascariasis	Schistosomiasis		
Toxocariasis			
Echinococcosis			
Enterobiasis			
Fascioliasis			
Hookworm			
Strongyloidiasis			
Tapeworms			
Trichinosis			
Trichuriasis			

* Also in the western United States
† Including the Caribbean

Table 2. Major Clinical Aspects of the Exotic Infections

General	*Fever.*—Smallpox; Yellow fever; Lassa fever; Plague; Shigellosis; Tuberculosis; Typhoid; Leishmaniasis, visceral; Malaria; Toxoplasmosis; Trypanosomiasis, African; Trypanosomiasis, American; Toxocariasis; Fascioliasis; Trichinosis
	Anemia.—Leishmaniasis, visceral; Malaria; Hookworm; Diphyllobothriasis
	Lymphadenopathy.—Plague; Toxoplasmosis; Trypanosomiasis, African; Trypanosomiasis, American; Filariases
	Eosinophilia.—Toxocariasis; Filariases; Fascioliasis; Schistosomiasis; Strongyloidiasis; Trichinosis
Chest	*Cough.*—Lassa fever; Plague; Tuberculosis; Paragonimiasis
Gut	*Abdominal pain.*—Shigellosis; Typhoid; Fascioliasis; Strongyloidiasis
	Diarrhea.—Cholera; Shigellosis; Amebiasis; Giardiasis; Strongyloidiasis; Trichinosis
	Dysentery.—Shigellosis; Amebiasis
Liver	*Jaundice.*—Hepatitis; Yellow fever
	Heptaomegaly.—Typhoid; Leishmaniasis, visceral; Toxocariasis; Echinococcosis; Fascioliasis; Schistosomiasis
	Splenomegaly.—Typhoid; Leishmaniasis, visceral; Malaria; Schistosomiasis
Skin	Smallpox; Leprosy; Leishmaniasis, cutaneous and muco-cutaneous; Enterobiasis; Onchocerciasis
Central Nervous System	Malaria; Toxoplasmosis; Trypanosomiasis, African; Schistosomiasis; Taeniasis solium

biguous step-by-step instructions for solving a clinical problem." [5] Our algorithms, which are presented as flow sheets with accompanying text, begin with a list of clinical observations suggesting the presence of a given exotic infection and then proceed through important diagnostic indicators such as geography, water contact, and insect bites. This descriptive information is followed by the recommendation of a single laboratory procedure or a linked sequence of tests in which the methodology is clearly delineated. When serologic tests are indicated, the most expeditious means by which they can be obtained is described. For treatment, only one drug regimen is usually recommended on the basis of a careful examination of all of the latest information.

The number of references appended to each article are few, ranging from 6 to 12. Most of these are citations to the original literature, and include the

Table 3. Sampling Sites for Diagnosis of the Exotic Infections

Blood	Hepatitis; Smallpox; Yellow fever; Lassa fever; Plague; Typhoid; Malaria; Trypanosomiasis, African; Trypanosomiasis, American; Filariases
Sputum	Plague; Tuberculosis; Paragonimiasis
Stool	Cholera; Shigellosis; Typhoid; Amebiasis; Giardiasis; Ascariasis; Flukes; Hookworm; Schistosomiasis; Strongyloidiasis; Tapeworms; Trichuriasis
Urine	Schistosomiasis
Skin	Smallpox; Leprosy; Leishmaniasis, cutaneous and muco-cutaneous; Enterobiasis; Onchocerciasis
Immunodiagnosis	*Serum.*—Hepatitis; Smallpox; Yellow fever; Lassa fever; Plague; Typhoid; Amebiasis; Malaria; Toxoplasmosis; Trypanosomiasis, American; Toxocariasis; Echinococcosis; Taeniasis solium (Cysticercosis); Trichinosis

most important papers of the past (not superseded by more recent efforts) as well as up-to-date information, particularly on diagnosis and treatment. Wherever possible only carefully controlled studies are cited, especially those concerning the usually uncontrolled descriptions of the clinical syndromes.

Three tables are presented as an aid to approaching the 26 articles concerned with particular infections. Table 1 presents the geographic aspects of the infections, revealing that they are either worldwide in distribution or are confined to Asia, Africa and/or Latin America. Table 2 lists the major signs and symptoms of the infections; it does not include the relatively minor, rare, or transient clinical aspects of the disease syndromes. Table 3 presents the major sampling sites for the diagnosis of the infection, via either demonstration of the infectious agent or sero-diagnosis.

This series of articles was prepared by 6 members and 3 adjunct members of the Division of Geographic Medicine of the Department of Medicine at Case Western Reserve University. They were all edited to a standard format by Drs. Kenneth S. Warren and Adel A. F. Mahmoud, who were themselves the senior authors of almost half of the articles. The Division of Geographic Medicine was particularly fitted to this task as all full-time members of the Division spend a significant portion of each year abroad doing clinical and epidemiological research on the infections described in the articles. Since the founding of the Division in 1974, with a generous grant from the Rockefeller Foundation, major programs have been carried on in Kenya, Ethiopia, Egypt, India, Vietnam, the Philippines, Guatemala, and St. Lucia.

The articles in this book were originally published in *The Journal of Infectious Diseases* in the period from May 1975 through October 1977. All of the older articles were revised on the basis of comments received from readers and brought up to date; this was accomplished in August and September 1977.

The editors and authors are extremely grateful to Dr. Edward H. Kass and to the editors and staff of *The Journal of Infectious Diseases* for their help and encouragement in this project. Susan Damsel, Project Coordinator of the Division of Geographic Medicine, was of particular help in organizing and indexing the articles for the present publication. We are also very grateful for the assistance of experts who perused several of the articles prior to initial publication: R. S. Guinto and R. Cellona (Leprosy); E. J. Gangarosa and R. B. Hornick (Shigellosis); R. B. Hornick (Typhoid fever); L. H. Miller (Malaria); J. S. Remington (Toxoplasmosis); and M. G. Schultz (Tapeworms).

References

1. U.S. Bureau of the Census. Statistical Abstract of the United States: (97th ed.) Washington, D.C., 1976.
2. Warren, K. S. Helminthic diseases endemic in the United States. Am. J. Trop. Med. Hyg. 23:723–30, 1974.
3. Neva, F. A. Protozoal diseases endemic in the United States. Am. J. Trop. Med. Hyg. 23:731–35, 1974.
4. Bowers, J. Z. and Cunnane, M. E. Teaching of parasitology and tropical medicine: A survey in 1973. Am. J. Trop. Med. Hyg. 23:791–92, 1974.
5. Ingelfinger, F. J. Algorithms, anyone? N. Engl. J. Med. 288:847–48, 1973.

Prevention of Exotic Diseases: Advice to Travelers

Exotic diseases are usually acquired by travelers to exotic places. Many of these diseases can be prevented by consultation with a physician prior to departure. To assess the risk of travel and to institute the necessary prophylactic measures, the physician must obtain the information shown in figure 1. Initially, the purpose of the trip should be ascertained, since the usual tourism and business travel on well-beaten paths tend to be associated with little risk. The destinations should be elicited since this information not only will aid in defining risk factors but also will permit the determination of specific prophylactic measures. Whether the travel will be confined to major urban areas or will include significant amounts of time in rural environments is important, as well as whether the accommodations will be luxurious hotels and lodges or local housing and tents. The duration of the trip is another factor essential to a determination of risk.

At one extreme, the low-risk traveler may be defined as the businessman staying in first-class hotels in the large cities of developed countries for short periods; these individuals rarely undergo any greater risk than those encountered in traveling in the United States. The opposite extreme is illustrated by the geologist living in tents or indigenous dwellings in the "bush" of the less-developed countries for long periods; he or she should be considered in the high-risk category and would benefit from a wide variety of prophylactic measures. These measures would include general advice on what to drink and eat and how to avoid insects, and specific measures involving immunizations, drugs, and information on special risks.

General Measures

Beverages. Drinking of untreated water is dangerous in most developing areas, as is ice prepared from that water, no matter what alcoholic beverage is added. Since most intestinal pathogens, including bacteria and amoebae, are heat-sensitive, water from a hot-water tap is relatively safe [1]; hepatitis A virus, however, appears to be only partially inactivated at these temperatures. Hot tea and coffee made from boiled water should be reasonably free of risk. Bottled beverages, with the exception of uncarbonated water, are usually safe. Fresh milk should be avoided in most tropical countries.

Food. Many of the precautions to be taken in developing areas are similar to those in the United States. Rare meats, including beef, can be more dangerous because pathogens other than *Trichinella spiralis* may be common (e.g., the beef and pork tapeworms). Raw or undercooked fresh-water fish can transmit liver flukes and tapeworms. Creamy desserts and rich sauces can act as growth media for the usual bacterial pathogens. Hot foods are usually safe. Peelable raw vegetables and fruits are relatively safe and are particularly innocuous if peeled by the eater. Lettuce is a particular offender because of the penchant of Americans for consuming it in large amounts, the practice of freshening the lettuce with any local source of water, the retention of infectious eggs, cysts, and bacteria by lettuce, and the difficulty of properly cleaning and disinfecting it.

Diarrhea. Prophylactic drugs for prevention of diarrhea are not recommended. Some of them such as iodochlorhydroxyquin (Entero-vioform), which is sold over the counter in many developing countries, has been associated with sub-acute myeloptic neuropathy, a condition that may lead to blindness [2]. If diarrhea without fever and blood occurs, it should be controlled largely by dietary discretion. Drugs that decrease intestinal motility probably should not be used as they can be dangerous in bacillary dysentery and are particularly contraindicated for children [3]. Liquid intake should be maintained for severe watery diarrhea. If the diarrhea persists for more than three days or is accompanied by fever or blood, a physician should be consulted. Lists of physicians can frequently be obtained from American embassies or consulates.

Insects. Unprotected individuals in tropical areas can suffer as many as 100,000 mosquito bites per year. Precautions should be taken, therefore, to minimize the number of bites; these measures include screening, use of bug bombs, mosquito netting, wearing of long-sleeved shirts and trousers (particularly in the evenings), and use of repellents, the best of which contain diethyltoluamide (e.g., OFF®, S. C.

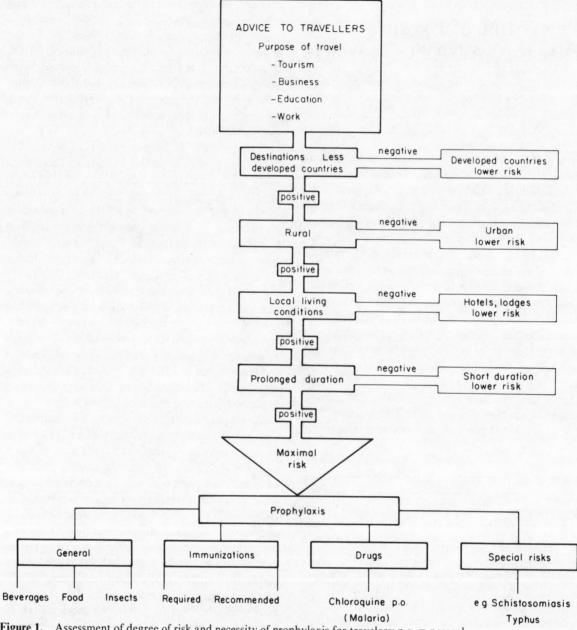

Figure 1. Assessment of degree of risk and necessity of prophylaxis for travelers; p.o. = peroral.

Johnson & Son, Racine, Wisc.). Similar precautions should be taken against other biting insects such as the tsetse fly and the blackfly. The common filth fly can transmit intestinal pathogens to food and drink, and such exposure should be minimized if possible.

Immunizations. General immunizations, such as those against polio and tetanus, should be up to date. The international requirements and individual health requirements for three major infectious agents (those of smallpox, yellow fever, and cholera) are

listed alphabetically by country in table 1 [4]. Because of a worldwide eradication campaign, smallpox is being transmitted at present in only a small area of East Africa (including Ethiopia and Somalia). Nevertheless, because of its communicability and pathogenicity, many countries still require vaccination. Revaccinations are required every three years. Yellow fever is also a highly fatal disease, and vaccination (required at 10-year intervals) is recommended for all travelers to endemic countries in Africa and

South America. Vaccination is also required by many countries for travelers who have been in endemic areas. Immunization against cholera may be required for travelers from or to endemic areas. This measure is not recommended as prophylaxis, however, because its efficacy is not high, and booster doses are required at six-month intervals.

Two other diseases of importance to travelers are not on the list of required prophylaxis for any country. Travelers at high risk should receive typhoid vaccine from which the useless paratyphoid components have now been removed. The vaccine does not afford complete protection but does reduce the risk of in-

fection, particularly when inocula are small. Since side effects are frequent, the minimal number of effective immunizations should be recommended. The results of one massive study reveal that a single primary dose is highly effective and remains so for seven years [5]. (The Center for Disease Control recommends two primary doses and boosters every three years [4].) For a partial protection against hepatitis A, travelers at high risk might be given immune serum globulin. For short-term travel, adults require 2 ml and, for longer-term travel, 5 ml repeated every six months. Immunization dosages for children may be found elsewhere [4].

Table 1. Necessity for prophylaxis against smallpox, yellow fever, cholera, and malaria before entry into various countries.

Country or area	Small pox	Yellow fever	Cholera	Malaria	Country or area	Small pox	Yellow fever	Cholera	Malaria
Afars and Issas	+	⊕	−	−	Chile	+	−	−	−
Afghanistan	+	−	−/+	+	China	+	−	+	?
Albania	−/+	−/+	−/+	−	Christmas Island	−/+	−/+	−/+	−
Algeria	−/+	−/+	−	+*	Colombia	+	⊕	−	+*
Angola	+	⊕	+	+	Comoro Archipelago	+	−	−	+
Antigua	−/+	−/+	−	−	Congo	+	⊕	−	+
Argentina	+	−	−	+**	Cook Island	−/+	−	−	−
Australia	−/+	−/+	−	−	Costa Rica	−/+	−	−	+*
Austria	−/+	−	−	−	Cuba	−/+	−/+	−	−
Azores	−/+	−/+	−	−	Cyprus	−/+	−/+	−	−
Bahamas	−/+	−/+	−	−	Czechoslovakia	−/+	−	−	−
Bahrain	+	−/+	−	+	Dahomey	−/+	⊕	−	+
Bangladesh	+	−/+	−	+	Denmark	−/+	−	−	−
Barbados	−/+	−/+	−	−	Dominica	−/+	−/+	−	−
Belgium	−/+	−	−	−	Dominican Republic	−/+	−	−	+**
Belize	+	−/+	−	+	Ecuador	+	⊕	−	+*
Bermuda	−/+	−	−	−	Egypt	+	−/+	−/+	+
Bolivia	+	⊕	−	+*	El Salvador	−/+	−/+	−	+
Botswana	+	−/+	−	+	Equatorial Guinea	+	⊕	−	+
Brazil	+	⊕	−	+**	Ethiopia	+	⊕	−	+
Brunei	+	−/+	−/+	−	Falkland Islands	+	−	−	−
Bulgaria	−/+	−	−	−	Faroe Island	−/+	−	−	−
Burma	+	−/+	−	+*	Fiji	−/+	−/+	−/+	−
Burundi	+	⊕	−	+	Finland	−/+	−	−	−
Cameroon	+	⊕	−	+	France	−/+	−	−	−
Canada	−/+	−	−	−	French Guiana	−/+	⊕	−	+
Canal Zone	+	−	−	−	French Polynesia (Tahiti)	+	−/+	−	−
Canary Islands	−/+	−	−	−	Gabon	+	⊕	−	+
Cape Verde Island	+	−/+	−/+	+					
Cayman Island	−/+	−	−	−					
Central African Republic	+	⊕	−	+					
Chad	+	⊕	−	+					

continued

Table 1 (*continued*).

Country or area	Small pox	Yellow fever	Cholera	Malaria	Country or area	Small pox	Yellow fever	Cholera	Malaria
Gambia	+	⊕	−	+	Luxembourg	−/+	−	−	−
Germany (East)	−/+	−	−	−	Macao	+	−/+	−	−
Germany (West)	−/+	−	−	−	Madagascar	+	−/+	−/+	+
Ghana	+	⊕	−	+	Madeira	−/+	−/+	−	−
Gibraltar	−/+	−	−	−	Malawi	+	−/+	+	+
Gilbert and Ellice Islands	+	−/+	−	−	Malaysia	+	−/+	−	+*
Greece	−/+	−/+	−	+**	Maldives	+	−/+	+	+*
Greenland	−/+	−	−	−	Mali	+	⊕	−/+	+
Grenada	−/+	−	−	−	Malta	−/+	−/+	−	−
Guadaloupe	−/+	−/+	−	−	Martinique	−/+	−/+	−	−
Guam	−/+	−	−	−	Mauritania	+	+	−	+
Guatemala	+	−	−	+*	Mauritius	+	−/+	−	−
Guernsey, Alderney, and Sark	−/+	−	−	−	Mexico	−/+	−/+	−	+*
Guinea	+	⊕	−	+	Monaco	−	−	−	−
Guinea-Bissau	+	⊕	−/+	+	Mongolia	+	−	−	−
Guyana	+	⊕	−	+*	Montserrat	+	−/+	−	−
Haiti	−/+	−/+	−	+*	Morocco	−/+	−	−	+
Honduras	+	−/+	−	+*	Mozambique	+	−/+	+	+
Hong Kong	+	−	−	−	Namibia	+	−/+	−	+
Hungary	−/+	−	−	−	Nauru	+	−/+	−/+	−
Iceland	−/+	−	−	−	Nepal	+	−/+	−	+
India	+	−/+	−/+	+	Netherlands	−/+	−	−	−
Indonesia	+	−/+	−	+	Netherlands Antilles	−/+	−/+	−	−
Iran	+	−/+	−/+	+	New Caledonia and dependencies	+	−/+	−	−
Iraq	+	−/+	−	+	New Guinea	+	−/+	+	+
Ireland	−/+	−	−	−	New Hebrides	−/+	−/+	−	+
Isle of Man	−/+	−	−	−	New Zealand	−/+	−	−	−
Israel	−/+	−	−	−	Nicaragua	+	−	−	+*
Italy	−/+	−	−/+	−	Niger	+	⊕	−	+
Ivory Coast	+	⊕	−	+	Nigeria	+	⊕	−	+
Jamaica	−/+	−/+	−	−	Norway	−/+	−	−	−
Japan	−/+	−	−	−	Oman	+	−/+	−/+	+
Jersey	−/+	−	−	−	Pacific Islands trust territories of U.S.	−/+	−	−	−
Jordan	+	−	−	+*	Pakistan	+	−/+	−/+	+
Kenya	+	⊕	−	+	Panama	+	⊕	+	+
Khmer Republic	+	−/+	−	+	Papua	+	−/+	+	+
Korea (Republic of)	+	−	−	+	Paraguay	+	−/+	−	+
Kuwait	+	−/+	−/+	−	Peru	+	⊕	−	+*
Laos	+	−/+	−/+	+	Philippines	+	−/+	−	+*
Lebanon	+	−/+	−	−	Pitcairn Island	−/+	−/+	−/+	−
Lesotho	+	−/+	−	−	Poland	−/+	−	−	−
Liberia	+	⊕	−	+	Portugal	−/+	−	−	−
Libyan Arab Republic	+	−/+	−/+	+**	Portuguese Timor	+	+	−	+
Liechtenstein	−/+	−	−	−	Puerto Rico	−/+	−	−	−
					Qatar	+	−/+	−/+	+
					Réunion	−/+	−/+	−	−

continued

Table 1 (*continued*).

Country or area	Small pox	Yellow fever	Cholera	Malaria	Country or area	Small pox	Yellow fever	Cholera	Malaria
Rhodesia	−/+	−/+	−	+	Swaziland	+	−/+	−/+	+
Romania	−/+	−	−	−	Sweden	−/+	−	−	−
Rwanda	+	⊕	−	+	Switzerland	−/+	−	−	−
Ryukyu Island	+	−/+	−/+	−	Syrian Arab Republic	+	−/+	−	+*
St. Helena	+	−	−/+	−	Taiwan	+	−	−/+	?
St. Kitts-Nevis-Anguilla	−/+	−/+	−	−	Tanzania	+	⊕	−	+
St. Lucia	−/+	−/+	−	−	Thailand	+	−/+	−	+*
St. Pierre and Miquelon	−/+	−	−	−	Togo	+	⊕	−	+
St. Vincent	−/+	−	−	−	Tonga	+	−/+	−	−
Samoa, American	−/+	−	−	−	Trinidad and Tobago	−/+	−/+	−	−
Samoa, Western	+	−/+	−	−	Tunisia	−/+	−/+	−	+*
Sao Tome and Principe	+	⊕	−	+	Turkey	−/+	−	−	+**
Saudi Arabia	+	−/+	+	+	Uganda	+	⊕	−	+
Senegal	+	⊕	−	+	U.S.S.R.	−/+	−	−	+**
Seychelles	+	−/+	+	−	United Arab Emirates	+	−/+	−	+
Sierra Leone	+	⊕	−	+	United Kingdom	−/+	−	−	−
Singapore	+	−/+	−	+*	United States	−/+	−/+	−	−
Solomon Island, British protectorate	+	−/+	−	+	Upper Volta	+	⊕	−	+
Somalia	+	⊕	−	+	Uruguay	+	−	−	−
South Africa	+	−/+	−	+	Venezuela	+	⊕	−	+*
Spain	−/+	−	−	−	Vietnam, South	+	−/+	−	+*
Spanish Sahara	−/+	−	−	−	Virgin Islands (U.S.)	−/+	−/+	−	−
Sri Lanka	+	−/+	−	+	Wake Island	−/+	−	−	−
Sudan	+	⊕	−	+	Yemen	+	−/+	−	+
Surinam	+	⊕	−	+	Yemen, Democratic	+	−/+	−	+
					Yugoslavia	−/+	−	−	−
					Zaire	+	⊕	−	+
					Zambia	+	−/+	−/+	+

NOTE. Key to symbols: (+) = necessary; (−) = unnecessary; (−/+) = unnecessary when traveling directly from the United States, but necessary when there is an outbreak in the United States or when traveling through countries where disease is endemic or an epidemic is occurring. (⊕) = yellow fever endemic. One asterisk indicates significant risk of malaria only in rural areas; two asterisks indicate significant risk of malaria in very few areas.

Drugs. It is worthy of strong emphasis that all travelers to areas in which malaria is transmitted (table 1) should receive the prophylactic drug chloroquine phosphate. Five hundred milligrams (300-mg base) should be taken orally once a week beginning one week prior to arrival, during the stay, and continuing six weeks after departure. This regimen will ensure protection against the potentially lethal *Plasmodium falciparum*. Delayed attacks with the less dangerous species of *Plasmodia* may occur within a few months or, rarely, years after return. In the event of persistent or recurrent fevers, the patient should be told to consult his physician and to advise him of exposure to malaria. Strains of *P. falciparum* that are resistant to chloroquine are found in Southeast Asia and northern South America, including Panama. Travelers to these areas should take chloroquine prophylaxis, but medical assistance should be sought immediately if a febrile illness occurs. Dosages for children may be found in reference 4.

Special Risks

The most common of the special-risk diseases is schistosomiasis, which is caused by a helminthic parasite widely spread throughout tropical regions.

The infective larvae of this parasite, which are found in freshwater streams, lakes, canals, etc., can rapidly penetrate unbroken skin. Travelers to most tropical areas should be warned against swimming in bodies of fresh water. Chlorinated swimming pools are safe, as is salt water.

Plague vaccine is advisable for persons traveling to the interior regions of Southeast Asia and those whose occupation brings them into contact with wild rodents in the epizootic areas of South America, Africa, and Asia. Epidemic louse-borne typhus exists only in highland areas where cold climates favor louse infestation. High-risk travelers to the remote highland areas of Asia should be immunized with the short-acting typhus vaccine.

Two inexpensive and reasonably concise sources of more detailed information are Health Information for International Travel 1977 [4] and Preservation of Personal Health in Warm Climates [6].

References

1. Neumann, H. H. Bacteriological safety of hot tapwater in developing countries. Public Health Rep. 84:812–814, 1969.
2. Anonymous. Traveler's warning: entero-vioform abroad. Med. Lett. Drugs Ther. 17:105–106, 1975.
3. Anonymous. Lomotil for diarrhea in children. Med. Lett. Drugs Ther. 17:104, 1975.
4. Center for Disease Control. Health information for international travel 1977, Morbidity and Mortality Weekly Rep. 26 (Suppl.):1–96, 1977.
5. Ashcroft, M. T., Singh, B., Nicholson, C. C., Ritchie, J. M., Sobryson, F., Williams, F. A seven-year field trial of two typhoid vaccines in Guyana. Lancet 2:1056–1059, 1967.
6. Preservation of personal health in warm climates. 7th ed. The Ross Institute of Tropical Hygiene, London, 1971. 102 p.

Acute Viral Hepatitis

Acute viral hepatitis is a significant public health problem in developing countries and remains a major cause of acute liver disease in the United States. It has been the cause of large outbreaks of jaundice throughout history and has been described by more than four dozen synonyms.

Classically, two major forms of hepatitis (A and B) have been delineated on the basis of clinical and epidemiologic evidence. The discovery of Australia antigen in serum [1], later called hepatitis B surface antigen, heralded an explosion of knowledge about the several infections that are called acute viral hepatitis. For example, the classical concepts of hepatitis A (infectious hepatitis) as an orally contracted disease and hepatitis B (serum hepatitis) as parenterally spread have been revised; hepatitis A and B may be spread by both routes. Moreover, seroepidemiologic data suggest that there is an additional type of hepatitis (hepatitis C?) and possibly more types [2].

Despite its high prevalence in many developing countries [3], hepatitis B does not appear to be a major source of infection for travelers. However, the high incidence of hepatitis A among American military personnel and Peace Corps volunteers abroad suggests that this virus is largely responsible for acute hepatitis in travelers returning to the United States.

Natural History and Epidemiology

Hepatitis A antigen is a 27-nm viruslike particle with a density of 1.32–1.40 g/cm^3 [4]. Antigen is detectable in the stool several days before acute hepatitis A infection becomes apparent and disappears before the clinical illness resolves [5]. The incubation period between exposure to infection and onset of clinical illness in hepatitis A is 15–50 days.

Hepatitis B surface antigen (HB$_s$ Ag) is a particle 22 nm in size that is incomplete viral protein coat. HB$_s$ Ag may be found in blood several weeks before the onset of clinically apparent hepatitis B and disappears in most persons at about the time clinical symptoms resolve. This antigen has been demonstrated in urine, stool, semen, tears, and saliva. About 10% of persons with acute hepatitis B become chronic carriers of HB$_s$ Ag. The Dane particle (44 nm in size), which is intact virus, is associated with hepatitis B core antigen (HB$_c$ Ag) and e antigen. The latter two antigens are most commonly detected during acute illness and are probably associated with viral replication. The incubation period for hepatitis B is 30–180 days.

There are three general sources of orally transmitted disease. First, hepatitis may be contracted from water supplies contaminated by human sewage. Second, food may become naturally contaminated, for example, oysters or clams may be cultivated in beds exposed to untreated sewage. When such foods are not cooked at temperatures sufficient to inactivate the virus, the virus remains infectious. Finally, food which is prepared or handled by persons who are infectious and practice poor hygiene may be the source of spread of disease to others. In this context the food is handled just before serving so that the status of cooking is irrelevant. The infectious source is probably stool. Intimate contact with infected persons also may result in transmission. Inoculation of contaminated blood either by transfusion or by contaminated medical, dental, or tattooing instruments is a possible source of infection.

The importance of animal reservoirs in the spread of hepatitis A and B is probably minimal. Hepatitis A antigen and HB$_s$ Ag have been associated with acute hepatitis in nonhuman primates, which in turn have been reported to be sources of spread of hepatitis among animal handlers and veterinarians. It is unlikely, however, that this is a major mode of infection for those who travel abroad or domestically. Blood-sucking insects also have been suspected of spreading hepatitis, but this mode appears to be an unlikely form of transmission [6].

Infection with hepatitis A is associated with the development of antibodies soon after the development of clinical illness, and such antibodies can be demonstrated by inhibition of immune adherence for as long as 10 years after active infection [7]. The presence of this antibody is associated with protection against subsequent infection with hepatitis A, but it is not protective for hepatitis B. Limited studies have demonstrated antibody to hepatitis A antigen in 45% of urban-dwelling Americans [8], whereas this antibody is present in the majority of persons living in hyperendemic regions of the world. This difference presumably explains the increased susceptibility of persons from areas of low prevalence traveling to hyperendemic areas and raises the possibility of the risk of large outbreaks in such unprotected populations. The prevalence of antibody to hepatitis A antigen is proportional to age and appears to be greater in areas of substandard environmental conditions [8]. Infection, with consequent development of antibody, occurs frequently in the absence of clinical signs of hepatitis A [8].

Antibodies against HB_s Ag (anti-HB_s) are detectable in serum late in the course of acute hepatitis B at the time that HB_s Ag disappears. They can be found in most persons at least three years after acute illness. Anti-HB_s is detectable in one-tenth to one-fourth of Americans, and its presence is associated with protection against hepatitis B in most persons. The asymptomatic carrier rate for HB_s Ag is 0.1% in the United States and appears to be inversely proportional to socioeconomic class. The carrier rate is considerably higher in the tropics.

Disease Syndromes

Infection with hepatitis A or B virus may result in a spectrum of clinical syndromes. Most persons do not have clinically apparent illness; the proportion of inapparent infection is estimated at 50%–90%. However, subclinical hepatitis is associated with elevations in levels of enzymes in serum. Clinical illness ranges from mild malaise to jaundice, prostration, nausea, vomiting, and diarrhea. Fever, when present, is usually mild. As with most viral diseases, the illness is usually milder in children than in adults.

In the majority of persons with clinically apparent disease, the infection usually resolves in two to six weeks, although either slowly resolving hepatitis or a posthepatitis syndrome consisting of lassitude and malaise is observed in a relatively small proportion of infected persons. The pathogenesis of these prolonged syndromes is unexplained but should not be confused with chronic active hepatitis. Chronic complications such as cirrhosis are probably more common after hepatitis B than they are with other types of acute viral hepatitis [9]. The extrahepatic manifestations of arthritis and rash, which are seen in as many as one-third of persons with hepatitis B, are probably not associated with hepatitis A.

Diagnosis

The diagnosis of acute viral hepatitis is outlined in figure 1. Malaise, nausea, and vomiting are frequent complaints at presentation. Since jaundice is present in <50% of all cases of acute viral hepatitis, its absence does not exclude the diagnosis. A history of known contact in the last six months with persons with acute hepatitis, ingestion of potentially infectious and inadequately cooked food (e.g., shellfish), blood transfusion, or travel where the disease is highly endemic supports the diagnosis. Other causes of acute hepatitis, such as allergic reactions to drugs, environmental toxins, or other infectious agents, must be ruled out by the appropriate history and laboratory tests. The absence of HB_s Ag throughout the course of infection suggests that the infectious agent is hepatitis A, but other etiologic agents may be involved.

Hepatomegaly is common, whereas splenomegaly occurs in the minority of cases. A rise in serum aspartate aminotransferase (SGOT) must be present for the diagnosis of acute hepatitis. The clinical and laboratory findings of hepatitis are so typical that liver biopsy rarely need be performed for confirmation of the diagnosis. This procedure should be reserved for cases in which it is necessary to exclude the possibility of hepatitis due to causes other than viral agents or when chronic hepatitis is suspected. If the levels of SGOT and bilirubin and the prothrombin time do not begin to approach normal three to six weeks after attainment of peak values, percutaneous liver biopsy can reasonably be performed, provided that studies of blood clotting permit such a procedure.

Management

Because management of hepatitis is generally expectant and supportive, hospitalization of the patient with uncomplicated hepatitis serves little medical purpose and unnecessarily exposes hospital personnel to infection. It can be assumed that the patient's usual intimate contacts will have been exposed to infection during the incubation period and early stages of the illness before the patient presents to the physician. Hospitalization may be reserved for the patient in whom the diagnosis is unclear, who will not maintain contact with the physician, who appears to be deteriorating, or who requires parenteral feeding.

Physical activity may be determined by the patient's own ability to be up and about. Moderate activity probably helps to maintain physical conditioning and may shorten the convalescent period.

When the illness is uncomplicated by signs of encephalopathy, dietary restrictions are unnecessary. Fat and protein content in the diet need not be limited. Indeed, a high fat content in the diet may increase palatability and, consequently, caloric intake. The appetite of patients with hepatitis will be so limited that they should be encouraged to eat anything that

is acceptable. Corticosteroids have no proven value in the management of acute viral hepatitis. Since preparation of food and sexual contact serve to spread hepatitis A and B, these activities should be limited during the acute illness, a dictum which is usually self-imposed because of malaise and fatigue. Careful washing of hands after using the bathroom should be observed. The patient should never donate blood after acute viral hepatitis.

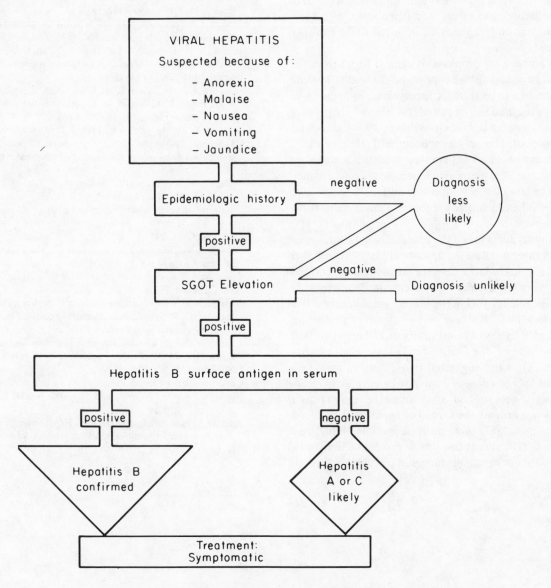

Figure 1. The progression to a diagnosis of viral hepatitis. SGOT = aspartate aminotransferase.

Prophylaxis

Until a vaccine is widely available, prophylaxis against clinically apparent hepatitis A can be achieved by passive immunization with standard, pooled immune serum globulin (ISG). ISG is not itself a source of hepatitis, and complications consequent to its administration are rare. When known exposure to hepatitis A has occurred, ISG in a dose of 2 ml for adults >100 pounds should be given as soon as possible since its effectiveness diminishes with increasing time between exposure and inoculation with ISG. Doses for children may be adjusted to 0.01 ml per pound.

The need for prophylaxis against hepatitis A for travelers going abroad depends on the level of hygiene in the area to be visited, the prevalence of hepatitis in that area, and the length of stay abroad [10]. Travelers who plan to visit cities only, stay in hotels, and drink bottled beverages probably need not receive ISG if their visit is for less than three months. On the other hand, travelers journeying to remote areas where they will be living under primitive conditions should receive ISG. When such trips are for less than three months, a single injection of 2 ml of ISG for adults of >100 pounds is adequate; if the exposure will be for longer than three months, the dose should be increased to 5 ml [10]. In the latter case, the dose should be repeated every six months during residence in these areas.

The role for ISG in the prevention of hepatitis B is controversial. Because of the apparent protection afforded by ISG against orally spread hepatitis B in some studies, the Center for Disease Control (Atlanta, Ga.) has suggested that currently manufactured ISG in a dose of 5 ml may be of value in clearcut exposures to fluid containing HB$_s$ Ag [11]. ISG does not prevent the spread of hepatitis B by blood transfusion. ISG preparations containing high titers of anti-HB$_s$ appear to be more protective than ordinary ISG in certain instances of intense exposure to HB$_s$ Ag [12] and are available for use in selected situations.

References

1. Blumberg, B. S., Alter, H. J., Visnich, S. A "new" antigen in leukemia sera. J.A.M.A. 191:541–546, 1965.
2. Villarejos, V. M., Visona, K. A., Eduarte, A. C. A., Provost, P. J., Hilleman, M. R. Evidence for viral hepatitis other than type A or type B among persons in Costa Rica. N. Engl. J. Med. 293:1350–1352, 1975.
3. Francis, T. I. Epidemiology of viral hepatitis B in the tropics. Bull. N.Y. Acad. Med. 51:501–507, 1975.
4. Purcell, R. H., Dienstag, J. L., Feinstone, S. M., Kapikian, A. Z. Relationship of hepatitis A antigen to viral hepatitis. Am. J. Med. Sci. 270:61–71, 1975.
5. Dienstag, J. L., Feinstone, S. M., Kapikian, A. Z., Purcell, R. H., Boggs, J. D., Conrad, M. E. Fecal shedding of hepatitis A antigen. Lancet 1:765–767, 1975.
6. Berquist, K. R., Maynard, J. E., Francy, D. B., Sheller, M. J., Schable, C. A. Experimental studies on the transmission of hepatitis B by mosquitoes. Am. J. Trop. Med. Hyg. 25:730–732, 1976.
7. Hilleman, M. R., Provost, P. J., Miller, W. J., Villarejos, V. M., Ittensohn, O. L., McAleer, W. J. Development and utilization of complement-fixation and immune adherence tests for human hepatitis A virus and antibody. Am. J. Med. Sci. 270:93–98, 1975.
8. Szmuness, W., Dienstag, J. L., Purcell, R. H., Harley, E. J., Stevens, C. E., Wong, D. C. Distribution of antibody to hepatitis A antigen in urban adult populations. N. Engl. J. Med. 295:755–759, 1976.
9. Redeker, A. G. Chronic viral hepatitis. *In* G. N. Vyas, H. A. Perkins, and R. Schmid [ed.]. Hepatitis and blood transfusion. Grune and Stratton, New York, 1972, p. 55–60.
10. Center for Disease Control. Health information for international travel 1975. Morbidity and Mortality Weekly Rep. 24(Suppl.):55–56, 1975.
11. Center for Disease Control. Perspective in the control of viral hepatitis, type B. Morbidity and Mortality Weekly Rep. 25(Suppl.):6, 1976.
12. Alter, H. J., Barker, L. F., Holland, P. V. Hepatitis B immune globulin: evaluation of clinical trials and rationale for usage. N. Engl. J. Med. 293:1093–1094, 1975.

Major Tropical Viral Infections: Smallpox, Yellow Fever, and Lassa Fever

Smallpox, yellow fever, and Lassa fever are easily spread viral infections that may be highly lethal and are essentially untreatable. Smallpox, once a major killer of mankind, has been virtually eradicated, and yellow fever is now well controlled through the use of a potent vaccine, while the newly discovered Lassa fever of West Africa represents an as yet uncontrolled threat.

Smallpox

Smallpox is one of the classical plagues of man. The etiologic agent of smallpox is the variola virus, one of the pox family of viruses, which includes a large number of related agents, e.g., cowpox, monkeypox, mousepox (ectromelia), etc. Infection with smallpox virus is highly contagious, disfiguring, potentially lethal, and essentially untreatable.

Smallpox was recognized as a disease entity in ancient times in Asia, the Middle East, and Africa. The infection spread to Europe and then to the New World as it was opened up to explorers and colonists from the Old World. In modern times, since Jennerian vaccination became widespread, smallpox was eradicated from most of North America and Western Europe and from Australia and New Zealand [1]. It has remained as a major disease in much of the rest of the world, however, with the greatest incidence in parts of Africa and the Indian subcontinent. In 1967 the World Health Organization inaugurated a worldwide campaign of vaccination with the explicit goal of eradicating smallpox. This ambitious program has had remarkable success. By the spring of 1977, smallpox was being reported only in Ethiopia, Somalia [2], and contiguous areas, and there is reason to believe that these last remaining foci will soon be eradicated [3].

If the present international effort to eradicate the disease is as successful as it seems to be, smallpox will soon be of historic interest only. Nonetheless, as long as the virus has not been eliminated, it is possible that a case can appear anywhere in the world, and it is critical that the diagnosis be made promptly if an epidemic is to be prevented.

Epidemiology. As there are no known animal reservoirs, persons infected with smallpox virus are the ultimate source of infection. Contact with infected individuals may be direct or indirect through utensils, clothing, or dust contaminated by the patient. A patient with smallpox must be considered infectious from the onset of the illness until the last scabs have dropped off. The virus can be transmitted early in the infection via the saliva and mucous secretions of the nose and later through the skin scabs. The smallpox virus is relatively resistant to environmental conditions; scabs wrapped in cotton and kept at 30 C–40 C maintained survival of the virus for up to six months, and at 20 C–25 C the virus was recovered after 17 months.

Unvaccinated persons of all ages and races are susceptible to smallpox. The recent outbreak of smallpox in London, England, which was started by an accidental laboratory infection, claimed the lives of two persons. It reminds us that as long as the possibility of the spread of infection exists, either from the few remaining foci in the horn of Africa or from accidents in research laboratories, an outbreak of smallpox is an ever-present danger.

A milder form of smallpox associated with a very low mortality, called variola minor or alastrim, has been observed during the present century. Although epidemiologically and clinically variola minor may differ from classical smallpox (variola major), no distinguishing features in the causative virus have been observed. Variola major and minor appear to be equally infectious, but the latter is more difficult to control because its presence is masked by the mildness of the disease.

Clinical features. The incubation period of smallpox is usually 12–13 days. The clinical illness begins with fever, malaise, and backache. Within two to four days, the characteristic rash appears, which then goes through a regular evolution of macule, papule, vesicle, pustule, and crust. The lesions all appear within 24–48 hr and have a typical centrifugal distribution. The initial lesions on the palms and soles, which feel like hard subcutaneous nodules, are almost pathognomonic. The timing and distribution of the lesions are helpful in differentiating smallpox from chickenpox (varicella): in the latter new lesions continue to appear for several days to a week and are more numerous on the trunk than on the face and extremities (centripetal) distribution. Furthermore, the smallpox vesicle is firm and multilocular, in contrast to the much more delicate, unilocular vesicle of chickenpox [1].

In the most severe cases of smallpox, the disease is almost always fatal as a result of pulmonary edema secondary to heart failure. In less severe forms, the mortality rate varies with the different clinical types of variola major. Thus, in one large outbreak the mortality rate was 6% in cases with discrete eruptions, 45% in cases with confluent eruptions, and 79% in those with hemorrhagic eruptions. The overall recorded mortality in that epidemic was 25%.

In alastrim or variola minor, the clinical features are similar to those of variola major with the exception that hermorrhagic or toxic cases occur only rarely, and consequently, there are few fatalities.

Diagnosis. An algorithm for the diagnosis and management of smallpox is shown in figure 1. The infection should be suspected in any febrile illness associated with skin eruptions. A geographic history is important because the patient or an acquaintance or relative may have been to an area where transmission of smallpox is still being reported. The possibility of accidental laboratory exposure should also be considered. The diagnosis of smallpox is less likely in a previously vaccinated individual, particularly if the last vaccination was within three years. The most important diagnostic step, however, is the clinical examination of the characteristics of the skin rash: the size and evolution of the lesions, their distribution, and evidence of single or progressive eruptions.

When the diagnosis of smallpox is considered likely, the patient should be brought immediately to the attention of the local public health authorities and the Center for Disease Control, Atlanta, Ga. so that the definitive diagnostic tests can be performed promptly by skilled personnel. Strict isolation procedures should be initiated, and all contacts should be identified. Specialized techniques are available for isolation of the virus from the blood before the eruptive stages. Smears of material obtained by scraping of the skin lesions can be stained by silver impregnation or fluorescent antibody methods, or the virus can be directly identified as a pox virus by electron microscopy. A negative finding on microscope examination of a smear from a person suspected of having smallpox should not be regarded as definitive, and isolation and identification of the virus in chick embryo or tissue culture should be attempted. Alterna-

tively, a rise in titers of antibody in the patient's sera indicates an active infection.

Management. There is no specific treatment for smallpox. Measures to alleviate symptoms are indicated whenever the need arises. Antibiotics are used to treat septic complications.

Prophylaxis. The principal protection against smallpox has been provided by vaccination. The great success of this vaccine has been its provision of solid protection against infection for three or more years. Furthermore, fatal disease is most unlikely in a person who has ever received even one successful inoculation.

For a good many years, the only justification for routine vaccination in the United States or much of Europe was to provide protection to those traveling to areas where smallpox was endemic or to prevent epidemic spread from imported cases. With the virtual elimination of the virus, the chances of infection have become so remote that many countries, including the United States, no longer require vaccination. Reactions to the vaccine are exceedingly rare; for example, of 900,000 individuals vaccinated in Wales in 1962, there were 26 cases of generalized vaccinia with one death and 17 cases of postvaccinal encephalitis with two deaths. Nevertheless, it was considered that the likelihood of a reaction to the vaccine, even though miniscule, contributed a greater risk than could be expected from the disease [4].

For some years to come, however, physicians and other health personnel who come in contact with large numbers of travelers should probably continue to be vaccinated, although even this procedure is no longer officially recommended in the United States, and a high level of vigilance should be maintained for imported cases. If smallpox is diagnosed, strict isolation of the case should be established, and all contacts should be vaccinated in order to contain the spread. The key to control is a high degree of suspicion, prompt reporting, rapid diagnosis, and immediate vaccination of the surrounding population.

Yellow Fever

Yellow fever is a disease of limited significance today, particularly in the Western Hemisphere. Historically, however, it was one of the important diseases of the tropical areas of Africa and the Americas. The origins of yellow fever are not known, but it is probable that

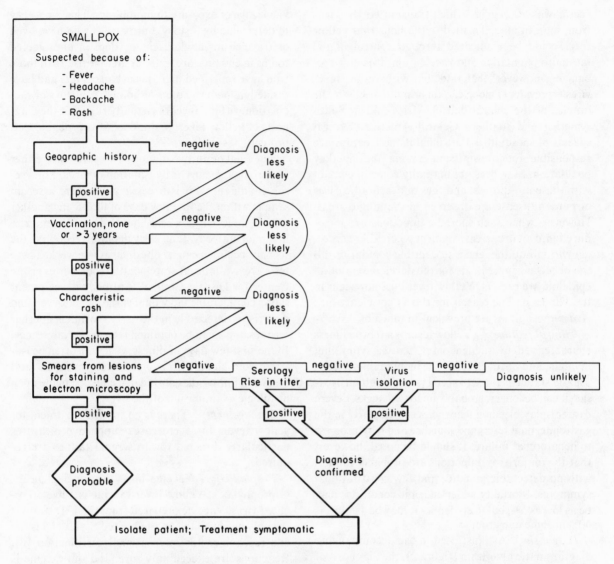

Figure 1.   The progression to a diagnosis of smallpox.

this disease occurred initially in Africa and was later introduced into the Americas. Yellow fever was one of the significant deterrents to immigration into the Caribbean and West Africa, and the story of its role in the disastrous attempt by the French to build a canal across Panama is known to every schoolchild. Epidemics occurred in urban areas and were not unusual well into the 19th century in seaports of the United States such as New York, Philadelphia, and New Orleans. Indeed, the last major epidemic in America was in New Orleans in 1905.

The etiologic agent of yellow fever is a group B arbovirus that is transmitted by mosquitoes of several genera. *Aedes aegypti* is the vector in urban settings.

With the recognition of the role of the mosquito in transmission and the introduction in 1932 of vaccination, it became possible to control the infection, and yellow fever is no longer the threat it once was. Nevertheless, because of its high fatality rate and the lack of any direct treatment, yellow fever remains an important risk to travelers in the rural areas of certain parts of Africa and Central and South America.

Epidemiology.   The principal epidemiologic fact concerning yellow fever is that natural transmission occurs only by means of the bite of an infected mosquito, as was conclusively proven by the report in 1911 of the U.S. Army Commission under Walter Reed in Cuba. For many years it was thought that the only vector was *A. aegypti* which transmitted the virus from man to man. This led to the hope that yellow fever could be eradicated through control of the mosquito population and vaccination. It is now recognized, however, that infection with yellow fever virus is prevalent among certain primate species in the jungles of the central belt of Africa and in South America and southern Central America. Several species of mosquitoes that inhabit the treetops are responsible for transmission among the monkey population. Man does not normally come in contact with these mosquitoes, and thus only sporadic cases of human disease are observed in the jungle areas. However, when such sporadic infections are introduced into an urban environment where there are *A. aegypti* mosquitoes and a susceptible population, all the necessary ingredients for the development of an epidemic are present. Yellow fever does not occur in the Far East. The reason for this is not clear since *Aedes* mosquitoes are prevalent in much of Asia.

Clinical features.   Yellow fever is a febrile illness characterized by sudden onset, nausea, vomiting, myalgia, and headache [5]. The incubation period is usually stated as three to six days, although on occasion it can be longer, probably up to two weeks. Severe cases display bleeding tendencies (particularly in the gastrointestinal tract) and jaundice and may progress to hepatorenal failure. It should be noted, however, that the majority of infections are probably milder, with no detectable jaundice and few constitutional symptoms. Mortality under endemic conditions may be as low as 5%, but in epidemics it may be as high as 40% in some age groups.

Diagnosis.   As illustrated in the accompanying diagrammatic algorithm (figure 2), the diagnosis of yellow fever is to be suspected in any person with a febrile illness associated with nausea, vomiting, and myalgia. The presence of jaundice, albuminuria, and gastrointestinal hemorrhage makes the diagnosis even more likely. The geographic history is paramount in importance, as the patient must either be resident in areas where yellow fever still occurs or have been a recent visitor to such an area. At present, yellow fever is endemic in the rural areas of northern South America and Panama; in Africa "jungle yellow fever" extends across the continent from the Sahara in the north through Tanzania-Zaire-Angola in the south. A listing by country can be found in "Advice to Travelers" (table 1). Laboratory infections are rare but have occurred. After a positive geographic history, the diagnosis is rendered more likely if there is

knowledge of exposure to mosquitoes. This is not easy to determine by history, but persons who have lived or traveled in jungle areas or slept in unprotected rooms in endemic areas are at greater risk than those who have remained in major urban centers and have resided in modern hotels or homes. A history of vaccination within 10 years virtually rules out the diagnosis of yellow fever, and indeed it is probable that protection is lifelong.

The final definitive diagnosis is established either by serologic means or by isolation of virus. For a serologic diagnosis it is necessary to secure a serum sample within the first few days of illness and another sample three to four weeks later to demonstrate a rise in titer of antibody. If an early diagnosis is desired, the second specimen can be obtained at one week. These tests are available at state health laboratories or the Center for Disease Control. Antibody development shows considerable individual variation, however, and if no rise is detectable in the early specimen, another serum sample can be obtained later in convalescence. In the first few days of illness, virus can often be isolated from blood by inoculation into mice. In fatal cases a definitive diagnosis can usually be made upon histologic examination of the liver.

Management.   There is no specific treatment for yellow fever. In severe cases supportive measures particularly directed towards renal failure are required.

Prophylaxis.   Vaccination is the principal means of prophylaxis. Yellow fever vaccine is a live attenuated virus. Vaccine prepared from the 17D strain is the only one available in the United States and is the one recognized for international certification [6]. Reactions are exceedingly rare, and the vaccine is highly effective. Duration of immunity is not known, although the international certificate is valid for 10 years, which is probably a conservative estimate. Another simple means of prophylaxis is prevention of mosquito bites via screening, netting, bug bombs, and repellents.

Lassa Fever

Lassa fever is a newly discovered viral infection in West Africa. This fever has emerged as a major public health problem because of the high case-fatality rate observed in hospitalized patients and its contagion for health care personnel. The infection is

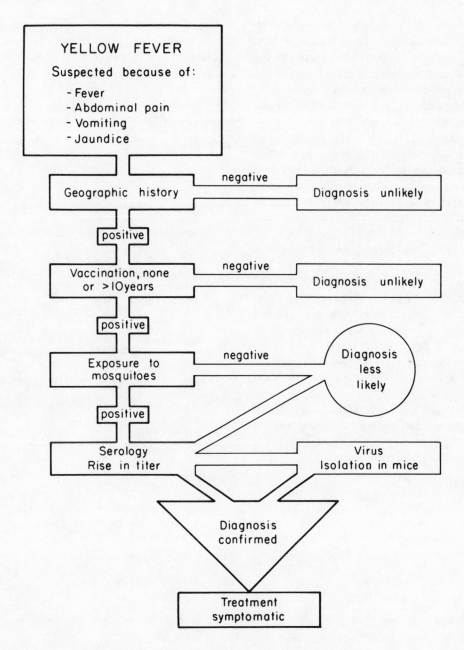

Figure 2. The progression to a diagnosis of yellow fever.

caused by a virus related morphologically and serologically to lymphocytic choriomeningitis virus and the hemorrhagic fever viruses of Argentina and Bolivia. A new taxonomic name of arenaviruses has been proposed for this group [7].

The first case of Lassa fever was observed in 1969 in a missionary nurse admitted to a hospital in Jos, Nigeria. She died, and two hospital employees were infected, one of whom also died. Since then, four epidemics have been recognized in Nigeria, Liberia, and Sierra Leone with a total of 101 cases and a mortality rate of 43% in hospitalized patients. Serologic surveys, however, indicate a wider distribution of the infection in West Africa with the possibility of inapparent subclinical infections. Individuals with severe febrile illnesses have been flown from Africa to Europe for treatment and were later found to have Lassa fever [8]. Laboratory-acquired infection has also been reported in an American investigator who worked with tissue cultures and mice infected with the Lassa virus. The few deaths that have occurred in Europe and the United States have drawn general attention to the problem, as serious questions have been raised about handling, transportation, and control of exotic infectious diseases.

Lassa virus has been found in nature in one animal species, the multimammate rat, *Mastomys natalensis,* but the mode of transmission to man is uncertain. Once established in humans, the infection seems to have spread from person to person in the hospital outbreaks and in the only known household outbreak in Sierra Leone.

Clinically, Lassa fever presents as a febrile illness associated with vomiting, cough, and pharyngitis. The definitive diagnosis can be made by demonstration of serum antibodies or by isolation of the virus; these studies should be attempted only in specially equipped laboratories such as the Center for Disease Control. If Lassa fever is suspected, the Center for Disease Control should be contacted immediately, and directions for processing and sending the samples should be obtained.

As the infection is highly contagious and may end fatally, special precautions must be instituted for handling of suspected individuals. Strict isolation of patients in specially equipped hospital units is nec-

essary. Therapy is largely supportive and symptomatic. Immune serum obtained from patients who have recovered from Lassa fever has been used for treatment and seems to have been successful in three of four cases.

References

1. Dixon, C. W. [ed.]. Smallpox. J. And A. Churchill, London, 1962, 512 p.
2. Smallpox—worldwide. Morbidity and Mortality Weekly Rep. 26: 83, 1977.
3. Henderson, D. A. The eradication of smallpox. Sci. Am. 235:25–33, 1976.
4. Lane, L. M., Ruben, F. L., Neff, J. M., Millar, J. D. Complications of smallpox vaccination, 1968. National surveillance in the United States. N. Engl. J. Med. 281:1201–1208, 1969.
5. Strode, G. K. [ed.]. Yellow fever. McGraw-Hill, New York, 1951. 710 p.
6. Center for Disease Control. Health information for international travel, 1977. Morbidity and Mortality Weekly Rep. 26 (Suppl.):1–96, 1977.
7. Casals, J. Arena viruses. Yale J. Biol. Med. 48:115–140, 1975.
8. Woodruff, A. W., Monath, T. P., Mahmoud, A. A. F., Pain, A. K., Morris, C. A. Lassa fever in Britain, Br. Med. J. 3: 616–617, 1973.

Cholera

Cholera is an acute illness caused by an enterotoxin elaborated in *Vibrio cholerae* that have colonized the small bowel of a susceptible individual. In the most severe form of cholera, there is rapid loss of fluid and electrolytes from the gastrointestinal tract, resulting in hypovolemic shock, metabolic acidosis, and, if untreated, death. Although the mortality rate may be extremely high in untreated cases, excellent therapeutic results can be obtained by prompt replacement of water and electrolytes by either the iv or the oral route [1].

Throughout the first six decades of the 20th century, cholera was largely confined to Asia, with the major endemic focus in the common delta of the Ganges and Brahmaputra rivers. The period 1961–1977 has witnessed a major pandemic spread of cholera from Indonesia westward through south and central Asia to western Europe and the entire African continent. Serious outbreaks of cholera occurred in Spain in the summer of 1972, in Italy in the summer of 1973, and in Guam in 1975, and isolated cases have been identified in travelers returning from these areas to most of the nations of western Europe. An isolated autochthonous case was identified in Galveston, Texas in 1974, and a single case occurred in a traveler to Canada in 1976.

Epidemiology

Man is the only documented natural host and victim of *V. cholerae*. Most epidemics of this disease appear to have been waterborne, and water plays the major role in the transmission of *V. cholerae* in rural areas where the disease is endemic. During large-scale epidemics, however, the direct contamination of food with infected excreta may also be important in the transmission of infection. Persons with mild or asymptomatic infections (contact carriers) may play a significant role in the dissemination of epidemic disease. In addition, a prolonged gallbladder carrier

state may develop in 3%–5% of adult patients convalescing from cholera caused by the biotype *eltor*, which has been responsible for the most recent pandemic. The gallbladder carrier state is more common in older convalescent patients and has never been observed in the pediatric group. The role of such convalescent carriers in the transmission of the disease has not been clarified.

In the endemic areas of Bangladesh and in West Bengal, cholera is predominantly a disease of children. Attack rates are 10 times greater in children one to five years old than in those older than 20 years [2]. When the disease spreads to previously uninvolved areas, the attack rates are initially at least as high in adults as in children. When cholera becomes endemic in new locations, however, as has occurred in the Philippines over the past 15 years, the endemic epidemiologic pattern develops, i.e., the disease becomes far more common in young children than in adults.

Disease Syndromes

Cholera results when a large number of viable *V. cholerae* are ingested, pass through the stomach, colonize the small bowel, and produce a potent protein enterotoxin. Because of the remarkable susceptibility of *V. cholerae* to gastric acid, an enormous number of microorganisms must be ingested to cause disease in a previously healthy individual. Studies in volunteers have indicated that intake of even 1.0×10^{10} organisms will not consistently produce clinical disease in individuals with intact gastric mucosa. If, however, gastric acid is neutralized by sodium bicarbonate, ingestion of 1.0×10^6 viable organisms produces clinical disease in roughly 50% of individuals [3]. Total or subtotal gastrectomy greatly increases susceptibility, as has been amply demonstrated by the recent experiences in Israel and Italy, where 20% and 35%, respectively, of cholera patients had undergone prior gastric surgery. It is interesting that the one individual who developed cholera in Galveston in 1974 had undergone such a procedure some years earlier.

Once the vibrios have colonized the small bowel, an enterotoxin with a molecular weight of 84,000 daltons is produced [4], binds rapidly, and apparently irreversibly, to small bowel epithelial cells and stimulates adenylate cyclase within these cells [4]. The resultant increase in intracellular levels of cyclic adenosine 3′:5′-monophosphate leads to the rapid secretion of water and electrolytes into the lumen of the small bowel. Stool from adults with cholera is nearly isotonic with plasma; the concentrations of sodium and chloride are slightly less than those of plasma, the bicarbonate concentration is approximately twice that of plasma, and the potassium concentration is three to five times that of plasma [5]. The action of the cholera enterotoxin on the small bowel results in no detectable morphologic damage to the mucosa [6].

The clinical onset of cholera is generally that of abrupt, painless, watery diarrhea. The volume of stool varies greatly; in the more severe cases, the first bowel movement may exceed 1,500 ml. At various intervals after the onset of diarrhea, vomiting ensues, which is also characteristically effortless and productive of clear watery material. In fulminant cases, severe muscle cramps, most commonly involving the gastrocnemius group, almost invariably develop. Prostration occurs at various intervals after the onset of symptoms and is in direct relationship to the magnitude of the fluid loss. When first seen by the physician, the typical cholera patient presents a characteristic appearance: collapsed, cyanotic, and with no palpable peripheral pulses, pinched facies, and scaphoid abdomen. Although the patient is usually conscious, the voice is very weak, high-pitched, and often nearly inaudible. Vital signs include tachycardia and varying degrees of tachypnea, hypopyrexia, and hypotension, often with no obtainable blood pressure. Heart sounds are faint or inaudible, and bowel sounds are hypoactive or entirely absent. Laboratory abnormalities are those that would be expected to result from the massive gastrointestinal loss of isotonic, alkaline, virtually protein-free fluid. These include increased specific gravity of plasma and whole blood, elevated level of plasma protein, decreased level of plasma bicarbonate, low arterial pH, normal level of plasma sodium, slightly increased level of plasma chloride, and moderately elevated level of plasma potassium [6]. Since the loss of bicarbonate is proportional to the volume of stool, the decrease in pH of whole blood is roughly proportional to the increase in plasma protein at all stages of the untreated disease. The illness may last from 12 hr to seven days, and later clinical manifestations depend on the adequacy of therapy. With fluid and electrolyte repletion, recovery is remarkably rapid. If therapy is inadequate, the mortality rate in seriously ill patients is often >50%. The important causes of death are hypovolemic shock, uncompensated metabolic acidosis, and uremia.

When renal failure occurs, the characteristic pathologic findings are those of acute tubular necrosis secondary to prolonged hypotension.

Diagnosis

The process involved in the diagnosis and management of cholera is illustrated in the accompanying algorithm (figure 1). If the diagnosis is suspected, appropriate replacement therapy, as indicated by the physical findings, should be initiated immediately. Although a cholera-like illness may be caused by organisms other than *V. cholerae* (notably enterotoxigenic *Escherichia coli*), the resulting metabolic abnormalities are similar, and the same therapeutic approach should be used in all such cases [7].

Following the initiation of appropriate therapy, a geographic history is of particular importance since the diagnosis of cholera is unlikely if the patient has not recently been in an area where cholera is known to be endemic or epidemic. Examination of stool specimens should then be performed. Since the cholera enterotoxin causes neither inflammation nor destruction of intestinal mucosa, leukocytes are not usually seen on microscopic examination of fresh stool from a person with cholera. This dictum is, however, not absolute, as cholera may occasionally be superimposed on other acute or chronic inflammatory bowel disease. Rapid tentative diagnosis can be made by direct observation of the characteristic rapid motility of the comma-shaped bacilli in fresh stool by dark-field microscopy; group and type-specific antisera clearly distinguish *V. cholerae* from other vibrios. Fluorescent miscroscopy using fluorescein-labeled type-specific antibody, when available, also provides a rapid and accurate means of identification [1].

The most reliable technique for definitive identification of *V. cholerae* consists of direct plating of the stool on thiosulfate-citrate-bile salt-sucrose (TCBS) agar upon which typical opaque yellow colonies appear in 18 hr. Final identification requires agglutination of the vibrios with group- or type-specific antisera and the demonstration of characteristic biochemical reactions.

Management

Successful therapy demands only prompt replacement of gastrointestinal losses of fluid and electrolytes. An

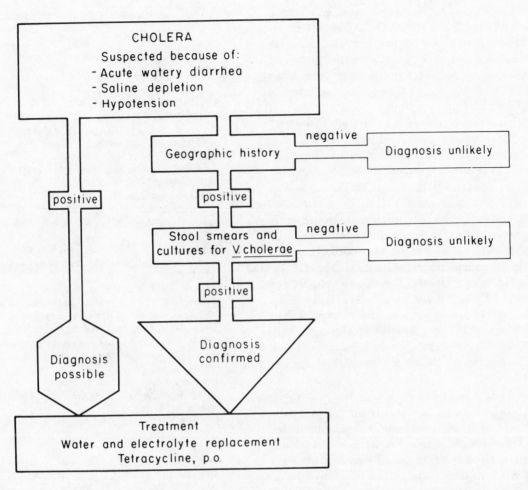

Figure 1. The progression to the diagnosis and management of cholera; p.o. = perorally.

iv solution, which is uniformly effective in adult patients, may be prepared by addition of 5 g of NaCl, 4 g of $NaHCO_3$, and 1 g of KCl to 1 liter of sterile distilled water [1]. The fluid should be infused rapidly (50–100 ml/min) until a strong radial pulse has been restored.

Subsequently, the same fluids should be infused in quantities equal to gastrointestinal losses. Close observation of the patient is mandatory during the acute phase of the illness, and overhydration should be avoided. An adult patient can lose as much as 1 liter of isotonic fluid/hr during the first 24 hr of the disease. Inadequate or delayed restoration of electrolyte losses results in a very high incidence of acute renal insufficiency. Serious hypokalemia is rare in the adult, and replacement of potassium can usually be carried out orally by giving approximately 15 meq of KCl for each liter of feces that is produced [5].

In children, complications are both more frequent and more severe [8]. The most serious include stupor, coma and convulsions (unique to pediatric patients), pulmonary edema, and cardiac arrhythmias that may occasionally lead to cardiac arrest. The central nervous system complications may be due to hypoglycemia, hypernatremia resulting from the iv administration of isotonic fluid to the pediatric patient, or cerebral edema, presumably secondary to rapid fluid shifts during the administration of iv fluids. Pulmonary edema may result if fluids are given iv at too rapid a rate, especially in the presence of severe metabolic acidosis. Serious cardiac arrhythmias may result from potassium depletion in children but rarely occur in adults with cholera. Each of these complications can be avoided by the careful administration of iv fluids that are especially designed to replace the fecal electrolyte losses of children with cholera. The following "diarrhea treatment solution," recommended by the World Health Organization, Geneva, Switzerland, has been used successfully to correct hypokalemia and hypoglycemia without provoking hypernatremia: sodium, 118 meq/liter; chloride, 83 meq/liter; potassium, 13 meq/liter; acetate, 48 meq/liter; and glucose; 50 mmol/liter [9]. Administration of this solution must be carefully monitored, with frequent ausculation of the lungs and inspection of venous filling in the neck to avoid overhydration. The outcome in pediatric cholera should be essentially as favorable as that in adults with the disease with an overall mortality rate of < 1% [1].

Peroral replacement of water and electrolytes is also remarkably effective in adults and in children who are alert, but glucose must be added to the solution to enhance its absorption [10, 11]. The oral glucose-electrolyte solution (1 liter of water plus 20 g of glucose, 3.5 g of NaCl, 2.5 g of $NaHCO_3$, and 1.5 g of KCl [11]) can be given in mild cases of cholera throughout the course of illness and is also satisfactory in the more severe cases, once the hypovolemic shock has been corrected by initial rapid iv fluid therapy [10].

Although adequate fluid therapy results in rapid physiologic recovery in virtually all patients with cholera, adjunctive treatment with antimicrobial drugs dramatically reduces the duration and volume of diarrhea and results in the early eradication of vibrios from the feces. Tetracycline in a daily dose of 40–50 mg/kg of body weight given orally in four equal portions every 6 hr for two days has been uniformly successful [12].

Immunization with two injections of 0.5 ml of the standard commercial vaccine (containing 1.0×10^{10} killed vibrios/ml) given at least one week apart provides 60%–80% protection for three to six months to adults in areas where cholera is endemic. At present, careful hygiene, particularly in relation to drinking water, provides the surest protection against cholera.

References

1. Barua, D., Burrows, W. [ed.]. Cholera. W. B. Saunders, Philadelphia, 1974. 458 p.
2. Mosley, W. H. The role of immunity in cholera. A review of epidemiological and serological studies. Tex. Rep. Biol. Med. 27:227–241, 1969.
3. Hornick, R. B., Music, S. I., Wenzel, R., Cash, R., Lebonati, J. P., Synder, M. J., Woodward, T. E. The Broad Street pump revisited: response of volunteers to ingested cholera vibrios. Bull. N.Y. Acad. Med. 47:1181–1191, 1971.
4. Finkelstein, R. A. Cholera. CRC Crit. Rev. Microbiol. 2:553–623, 1973.
5. Carpenter, C. C. J., Mitra, P. P., Sack, R. B. Clinical studies in Asiatic cholera, parts I–VI. Bull. Johns Hopkins Hosp. 118:165–245, 1966.
6. Gangarosa, E. J., Beisel, W. R., Benyajati, C., Sprinz, H., Piyaratin, P. The nature of the gastrointestinal lesion in Asiatic cholera and its relation to pathogenesis: a biopsy study. Am. J. Trop. Med. Hyg. 9:125–135, 1960.
7. Sack, R. B. Human diarrheal disease caused by enterotoxigenic Escherichia coli. Annu. Rev. Microbiol. 29:333–353, 1975.
8. Hirschhorn, N., Lindenbaum, J., Greenough, W. B., Alam, S. M. Hypoglycemia in children with acute diarrhea. Lancet 2:128–132, 1966.
9. Griffith, L. S. C., Fresh, J. W., Watten, R. H., Villaroman, M. P. Electrolyte replacement in paediatric cholera. Lancet 1:1197–1199, 1967.
10. Pierce, N. F., Sack, R. B., Mitra, R. C., Banwell, J. G., Brigham, K. L., Fedson, D. S., Mondal, A. Replacement of water and electrolyte losses in cholera by an oral glucose-electrolyte solution. Ann. Intern. Med. 70:1173–1181, 1969.
11. Mahalanabis, D., Choudhuri, A. B., Bagchi, N. G., Bhattacharya, A. K., Simpson, T. W. Oral fluid therapy of cholera among Bangladesh refugees. Johns Hopkins Med. J. 132:197–205, 1973.
12. Wallace, C. K., Anderson, P. N., Brown, T. C., Khanra, S. R., Lewis, G. W., Pierce, N. F., Sanyal, S. N., Segre, G. V., Waldman, R. H. Optimal antibiotic therapy in cholera. Bull. W.H.O. 39:239–245, 1968.

Leprosy

Leprosy is a chronic bacterial infection of man that is caused by *Mycobacterium leprae*. Skin and peripheral nerves are primarily involved, but other tissues, especially the eyes, mucosa of the upper respiratory tract, muscle, and testes, may be affected [1]. The clinical pattern varies depending upon the reaction of the host to the organism. An individual patient may be anywhere on a spectrum between the two polar types of leprosy, lepromatous and tuberculoid. Lepromatous leprosy is characterized by enormous bacterial growth concomitant with gross impairment of cell-mediated immunity, whereas patients with tuberculoid leprosy have an intense lymphocytic reaction and organisms can be found only rarely [2]. The immunological and clinical status is not necessarily static since patients may move toward either pole during the course of the disease.

It is estimated that there are 15 million patients with leprosy throughout the world. The infection is most prevalent in Africa, South and Southeast Asia, and parts of South America. A prevalence of more than five affected persons per 1,000 population is common in endemic areas, and the highest levels are seen in tropical Africa where 20–50 persons in every 1,000 may be afflicted. In the United States, 100–150 new cases are reported every year; most of these cases are imported, particularly by Puerto Ricans, Mexicans, and immigrants from Asia. Autochthonous infections are especially found in California, Texas, and Hawaii [3].

Epidemiology

Leprosy occurs slightly more frequently in males than in females. Although the disease appears at any age, teenagers and young adults are most commonly affected. The epidemiological factors that determine the distribution and prevalence of the infection are not well understood. As far as is known, man is the only natural host for *M. leprae*. The organism is an obli-

gate intracellular parasite, and the bacteria multiply at the very slow rate of every three to four weeks within mononuclear phagocytes, especially the histiocytes of the skin and Schwann cells of the nerves. Patients with lepromatous leprosy are the most likely source of infection. The bacilli are shed in nasal secretions and discharges from ulcers. The skin is the most likely portal of entry, but the possibility of infection via the respiratory tract has not been excluded. The usual incubation period is about two to four years, although periods of as short as three months and as long as 40 years have been reported.

It is not known which segment of the population is most susceptible to infection with *M. leprae*, why many patients heal spontaneously, or why some individuals develop lepromatous disease and others develop tuberculoid leprosy. There are geographical variations in the frequency of the different types of leprosy; for example, lepromatous leprosy is relatively more common in Eastern Asia than it is in India or Africa. It has been suggested that this variation is due to differences in genetically determined susceptibility, but different strains of the organism or variations in exposure patterns may be factors.

In most areas where leprosy is endemic, there is slow spread of infection. Cases tend to be clustered in families or villages, and the risk of contracting the disease is greatest among those who live for prolonged periods in close contact with infectious individuals. Nevertheless, one-half to two-thirds of patients have had either no known contact with infectious persons or apparently only transient exposure. It has been estimated that three-quarters of all patients with an early, solitary lesion heal spontaneously.

Clinical Syndromes

The earliest sign of leprosy is commonly an asymptomatic, ill-defined hypopigmented macule several centimeters in diameter that is often found on the trunk or upper aspects of the limbs. There may be mild impairment of sensation. Many of these lesions, which are classified as indeterminate leprosy, disappear completely. In some patients, however, the condition progresses into one of the patterns that make up the spectrum of disease in leprosy; classification of the infection depends on the degree to which cell-mediated immunity develops [4].

Lepromatous leprosy. Lepromatous leprosy has an insidious onset and often has a steady downhill course that results in multiple organ involvement and death in the untreated patient. The early skin lesions are bilaterallly symmetrical patches of diffuse infiltration with a shiny, erythematous surface. They are not anesthetic and often not hypopigmented. In untreated cases the lesions coalesce giving the skin a full, waxy appearance. Thickening is most marked on the face, especially the forehead, eyebrows, nose, malar surfaces, and earlobes. The thickened skin may develop into folds (leonine facies), and nodules may appear which are raised centrally and slope off imperceptibly. The eyebrows and eyelashes may be lost. In patients whose disease falls between borderline and lepromatous leprosy, the lesions are similar except that they are not absolutely symmetrical, and areas of normal skin are seen between the lesions; papules and nodules thus may stand out.

Gradual destruction of the small peripheral nerves in lepromatous leprosy produces a symmetrical anesthesia, beginning on the extensor surfaces of the forearms, hands, legs, and feet and slowly spreading to the trunk and face. In the later stages, the large nerve trunks become involved with an end result similar to that seen in tuberculoid leprosy. Nerve damage and its resultant trauma and secondary infection, together with bacillary infiltration of the skin, muscle, and medulla of the phalanges, leads to swollen and tense hands and feet, thin brittle nails, and gradual symmetrical shortening of the fingers and toes.

Involvement of the mucosa of the nose and throat may occur leading to nasal stuffiness, ulceration of the nasal septum, collapse of the nasal bridge, hoarseness, and laryngeal obstruction. Lepromatous infiltration of the eye may cause a punctate keratitis, conjuctival nodules, or iridocyclitis. Death may result from respiratory obstruction, inanition, renal failure, or secondary infection, especially tuberculosis, tetanus, or pyogenic infections of wounds of the anesthetic limbs.

Borderline leprosy. Many skin lesions with a tendency to symmetry are found in borderline leprosy. There is great variety in size, shape, and marginal definition. The lesions are reddish in color, often with a waxy surface, and may be hypoesthetic. A widespread, severe neuropathy, as described below, usually occurs.

Tuberculoid leprosy. The skin lesions either are plaques or have a raised edge with a flat, healing center; they are few in number and vary in size from 3 to 30 cm. The lesions are asymmetrical, hypopig-

mented, anesthetic, hairless, and dry and have a well-defined margin. The lesions in patients whose disease falls between tuberculoid and borderline leprosy are similar, except that the marginal definition is less absolute (there are often small satellite lesions) and there may be more of them.

One or more large peripheral nerves or any cutaneous nerve in association with a skin lesion may be palpable; nerve involvement is much more severe in patients with some features of borderline leprosy. Sensory, motor, and autonomic functions are involved, but usually the sensory component, first of pain and then of touch, is most affected. Anesthesia results in the most severe complications as excessive forces are applied to the tissues causing ischemia and injury. Autonomic dysfunction produces a warm, dry skin which becomes hard and brittle with fissuring. Secondary infection commonly occurs and causes further tissue damage. All of these factors lead to plantar ulceration, fractures, osteomyelitis, and irreversible distortion of the hands and feet.

Motor nerve involvement is often patchy. Partial paralysis of the hand results from damage to the ulnar nerve; when the median nerve is involved as well, a total "claw" hand develops. At first the hand is mobile, but if contractures develop the hand becomes fixed. Involvement of the radial nerve produces wristdrop, and that of the lateral popliteal nerve, footdrop. Damage to the posterior tibial nerve results in anesthesia of the sole of the foot and paralysis of the musculature that leads to clawing of the toes and collapse of the arches. Facial nerve palsy causes inability to close the eyelids, and involvement of the trigeminal nerve produces anesthesia of the cornea and conjunctiva. These features may result in ectropion, traumatic keratitis, corneal ulceration, and all of their attendant complications.

Reactions. Reactions are characterized by the appearance of symptoms and signs of acute inflammation of the lesions. Two types of reaction may complicate the course of leprosy.

(*1*) Lepra reactions tend to occur in patients with borderline disease and are usually accompanied by a change in cellular immunity. These reactions may occur spontaneously or be precipitated by the introduction or interruption of antibacterial therapy. The skin lesions become swollen, red, and edematous. The nerves swell rapidly and may be very tender and extremely painful. Loss of sensorimotor function is rapid and may be permanent. Fever, malaise, and prostration are common and may last for weeks or months.

The reactions tend to recur, and steady deterioration may culminate in death.

(*2*) Erythema nodosum leprosum, which usually occurs in patients with lepromatous leprosy, may arise spontaneously but is often precipitated by treatment. It results from immune-complex deposition in the tissues and is characterized by the appearance of painful, red, dome-shaped skin nodules which may ulcerate. The nodules usually last for a few days and are often succeeded by a crop of new ones. Chronic erythema nodosum leprosum produces a brawny induration, commonly on the extensor surfaces of the limbs. Iritis, dactylitis, and nephritis may develop.

Diagnosis

An algorithm for the diagnosis and management of

leprosy is shown in figure 1. Leprosy may be suspected because of skin lesions, numbness, anesthesia, muscle weakness, or blurring of vision. Thickened nerves may be noticed on clinical examination.

A geographic history is important since the diagnosis is unlikely if the patient has not lived in an area where leprosy is endemic. Residence in an endemic area and prolonged contact with patients with leprosy, particularly family members with lepromatous leprosy, greatly increases the likelihood of the diagnosis.

Whether or not a bacteriologically confirmed diagnosis will be made depends upon the type of leprosy: bacilli abound in lepromatous leprosy but are extremely rare in tuberculoid leprosy. Nevertheless, bacilli should be sought in slit skin smears from all patients. Smears are taken from suspected lesions as well as from the forehead, earlobes, chin, extensor surfaces of the forearms, buttocks and trunk. The skin

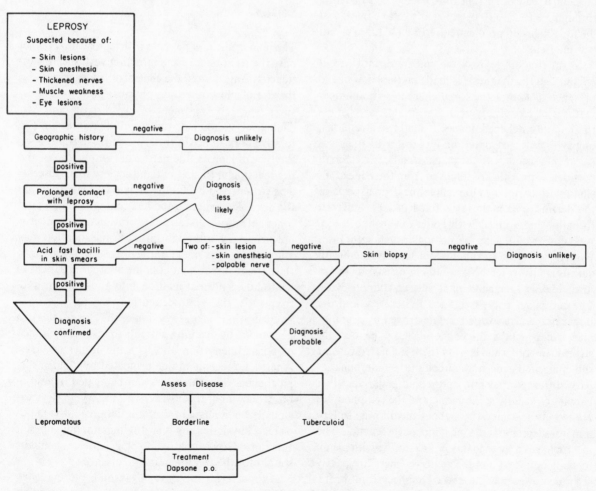

Figure 1.   The progression to the diagnosis and treatment of leprosy; p.o. = perorally.

is pinched tightly between the forefinger and the thumb to prevent blood flow, a fine incision is made in the dermis with a scalpel, and the cut surface of the tissue is scraped. The fluid, which must not be bloody, is smeared on a slide and allowed to dry. Smears can also be made of nasal discharges or washings. The slides are passed through a flame several times and stained by Ziehl-Neelsen's method in which they are covered with carbol-fuchsin (1 g of basic fuchsin, 10 ml of 95% ethanol, and 90 ml of 5% phenol) for 20 min, decolorized with acid-alcohol (30 ml of distilled water, 69 ml of 95% ethanol, and 1 ml of concentrated hydrochloric acid), and counterstained with methylene blue (0.3 g of methylene blue, 30 ml of 95% ethanol, and 70 ml of distilled water) for 1 min. The slides are then examined by means of an oil immersion lens at a magnification of × 100; the bacilli can be seen as red rods against a blue background. The density of bacilli is recorded as the bacteriological index on a scale of 1+ (one to 10 bacilli per 100 fields) through 3+ (one to 10 bacilli in an average field) and 5+ (> 100 bacilli per one field) to 6+ (> 1,000 bacilli per one field).

In tuberculoid leprosy the smears do not reveal bacilli, and the diagnosis is made on the basis of the presence of two of the three characteristic clinical features of leprosy: typical skin lesions, skin anesthesia, and thickened nerves. If doubt still remains, biopsy of affected tissue may reveal a histological picture consistent with the diagnosis of leprosy. Small portions of the skin are removed from the edge of lesions, with care taken to include the deep aspects of the dermis. The material is fixed in 10% buffered formalin and stained with hematoxylin and eosin. Acid-fast bacilli may be demonstrated with Fite-Faraco stain [5]. In tuberculoid leprosy the entire dermis is infiltrated by granulomas consisting of epithelioid cells, Langhan's giant cells, and lymphocytes. The cutaneous nerve twigs are obliterated, and the larger nerves are swollen and destroyed by granulomas. Acid-fast bacilli cannot usually be demonstrated. In borderline leprosy there is a narrow, clear sub-epidermal zone, and, although the macrophages have differentiated into epithelioid cells, acid-fast bacilli are usually seen readily and the lymphocytes are loosely scattered throughout the dermis. In lepromatous leprosy there is no lymphocyte reaction. The macrophages appear foamy or are stuffed with bacilli forming acid-fast globi. The nerve fibers are partly separated by edema, there is no lymphocytic infiltrate, and acid-fast bacilli are seen in the cytoplasm of the enlarged Schwann cells.

If the diagnosis is bacteriologically confirmed or considered probable on the basis of the clinical features and histology, the type of leprosy [4] is determined by correlation of the clinical features characteristic of each type of leprosy with the bacteriological index, the histological picture, and the result of the lepromin test (table 1). This test is not diagnostic of leprosy but is useful in grading the disease. Lepromin may be obtained from the Chief Medical Officer, Leprosy, Division of Communicable Diseases, World Health Organization, Geneva 27, Switzerland. Lepromin (0.1 ml) is injected intradermally, and the site is examined after 72 hr for a tuberculin-type response and after four weeks for a nodule. Observation of the latter is more reliable, and the result is considered positive if there is a reaction of ≥5 mm in diameter.

Management

The management of patients with leprosy involves not only the treatment of the infection with specific antibacterial agents and the control of reactions but also the use of physiotherapy, physical preventive measures, surgery, treatment of eye disease, and psychological, vocational, and social rehabilitation. The relative importance of these measures depends upon the type of leprosy, the nature of complications, and the reaction of the patient and society to his disease. The patient and his family should be reassured that the disease is treatable and less contagious than most other infectious diseases. Institutional treatment is not necessary, although initial hospitalization may allow better assessment of the disease and training of the patient. Treatment at home allows the patient to continue his normal relationships and contacts and, frequently, the same occupation.

Ulceration and destruction of the extremities can be avoided by teaching patients to respect their lack of normal sensation and to avoid injurious tasks. Anesthetic feet should be protected by molded surgical shoes. Plantar ulcers can be healed by immobilization, and reconstructive surgery may occasionally be indicated for motor deficits of the hands or feet. Physiotherapy is useful in maintaining motor functions. Expert ophthalmological advice should be sought for the treatment of eye disease.

Antibacterial therapy. Dapsone, the mainstay of drug treatment for leprosy, is cheap, safe, and effective [6]. The dose is built up slowly to minimize the

Table 1. Clinical, bacteriological, pathological, and immunological features of the different types of leprosy.

Feature	Lepromatous	Borderline lepromatous	Borderline	Borderline tuberculoid	Tuberculoid
Skin lesions					
Number	Very many	Many	Moderate numbers	Few to moderate numbers	One to three
Nature	Diffuse, waxy, thickening	Diffuse, papules	Polymorphic	Incompletely demarcated, hypopigmented	Well-demarcated, hypopigmented
Symmetry	Symmetrical	Slightly symmetrical	Asymmetrical	Asymmetrical	Asymmetrical
Anesthesia	None	Slight	Moderate	Marked	Marked
Nerve lesions					
Palpable nerves	Uncommon	Occasional	Common	Common	Occasional
Sensorimotor dysfunction	Symmetrical	Mixed	Asymmetrical	Asymmetrical	Asymmetrical
Bacterial index*	5–6+	3–5+	2–4+	1–2+	0
Skin histology					
Epithelioid cells	0	0	+	++	++
Foam cells	++	+	0	0	0
Lymphocytes	±	+	+	++	+++
Subepidermal infiltration	0	0	0	±	+
Dermal nerve destruction	0	±	+	++	+++
Lepromin test result	0	0	±	+	+++
Reactions					
Lepra	0	+	++	+	0
Erythema nodosum leprosum	++	+	0	0	0

NOTE.   +++ = many or severe; ++ = moderate number or moderate; + = few or slight; ± = questionable; 0 = not present.

* The density of bacilli is recorded on a scale of 1+ (one to 10 bacilli per 100 fields) through 3+ (one to 10 bacilli in an average field) and 5+ (>100 baccilli per one field) to 6+ (>1,000 bacilli per one field).

frequency of reactions. The initial dose is 25 mg weekly, and the dose is increased by 25 mg every two weeks until a final dose of 50 mg daily for adults is reached. Patients with lepromatous leprosy are usually treated throughout their lives, particularly if they remain lepromin-negative. Patients with other forms of leprosy should be treated until there are no signs of disease activity plus at least that length of time of treatment again; as a rough guide, 10 years of treatment for borderline and about three to five years for tuberculoid leprosy are required. Side effects are few although rashes, hypermelanosis, or mild hemolysis, especially in individuals with glucose-6-phosphate dehydrogenase deficiency, may occur. More importantly, lepra reactions and erythema nodosum leprosum may be precipitated. Resistance to dapsone may emerge in patients with lepromatous leprosy who have been treated for 10–20 years, especially if the drug has been taken irregularly. Rifampicin in a dose of 600 mg daily may be used if the patient is intolerant of dapsone or if dapsone resistance develops.

Treatment of reactions. Early diagnosis and treatment of reactional states will prevent much nerve and eye damage. Minor reactions may be controlled with 600 mg of aspirin every 4 hr. Severe reactions with threatening paralysis or anesthesia, iritis, orchitis, severe skin ulceration, or systemic disturbance require rapid control with 60 mg of prednisolone daily in divided doses. Whenever possible, the steroids should be slowly withdrawn during a period of four to eight weeks. If steroids cannot be withdrawn or patients are troubled by continuous erythema nodosum leprosum, the patients should be referred to a center that specializes in the treatment of leprosy; a physician at such a center may substitute clofazimine, which is both antibacterial and antiinflammatory, for dapsone.

Specialist Centers in the United States

When difficulties in the diagnosis or management of patients with suspected or proven leprosy are encountered, help may be obtained from the following specialist centers in the United States: U.S. Public Health Service Hospital, Carville, La. 70721 (telephone 504-642-7771); U.S. Public Health Service Hospital, 2 Fourteenth Avenue, San Francisco, Calif. 94118; U.S. Public Health Service Hospital, Bay Street at Vanderbilt Avenue, Staten Island, N.Y. 10304; Molokai General Hospital, Box 408, Maui County, Hawaii 96748.

References

1. Bryceson, A., Pfaltzgraff, R. E. Leprosy for students of medicine. Churchill Livingstone, Edinburgh, 1973. 152 p.
2. Turk, J. L., Bryceson, A. D. M. Immunological phenomena in leprosy and related diseases. Adv. Immunol. 13:209–266, 1971.
3. Center for Disease Control. Leprosy—United States, Puerto Rico. Morbidity and Mortality Weekly Rep. 28(20):163, May 28, 1976.
4. Ridley, D. S., Jopling, W. H. Classification of leprosy according to immunity, a five group system. Int. J. Lepr. 34:255–273, 1966.
5. Manual of histological and special staining technics of the Armed Forces Institute of Pathology. 2nd ed. McGraw Hill, New York, 1960, p. 177.
6. Browne, S. G. The drug treatment of leprosy. Trans. R. Soc. Trop. Med. Hyg. 61:265–271, 1967.

Plague

Plague is an acute bacterial infection of man caused by *Yersinia pestis*. The natural reservoirs of the organism are predominantly urban and sylvatic rodents, and it is transmitted among animals and occasionally to man by bites of infected fleas. Plague has a cosmopolitan distribution with significant foci of infection in the Americas, Africa, and Asia. *Y. pestis* has caused devastating pandemics throughout history with high mortality rates, in which pneumonic man-to-man transmission has occurred in addition to the usual flea-to-man spread. Today, in the United States, urban plague carried by rats has been eliminated, but sylvatic plague persists in rodents and other mammals of rural areas in the southwestern states with occasional transmission to man. The most common clinical form is acute regional lymphadenitis, called bubonic plague. Less common forms include septicemic, pneumonic, and meningeal plague. Mortality is high in untreated patients, but antibiotic treatment with streptomycin administered early in the course of the disease markedly reduces fatalities.

Epidemiology

The causative agent, *Y. pestis,* belongs to the family of bacteria Enterobacteriaceae. It is an aerobic Gram-negative bacillus which is readily cultured in broth or agar media with an optimal growth rate at 28 C. *Y. pestis* is well adapted to a variety of mammalian hosts in which it maintains itself by flea transmission. The most important reservoirs worldwide are the rats *Rattus rattus* and *Rattus norvegicus*. In the United States sylvatic rodents and other mammals are the major reservoirs of the plague bacillus. These include prairie dogs, squirrels, chipmunks, field mice, wood rats, rabbits, coyotes, and bobcats [1].

Human infection with *Y. pestis* is usually due to the bite of infected animal fleas. In the United States, a significant proportion of cases of plague occur as a result of hunters handling infected animal tissues. Man is an accidental host and plays no role in the maintenance of plague in nature. Epidemics are usually preceded by and accompanied by epizootics in rodents, which may die in large numbers. Less commonly, epidemics of pneumonic plague may be propagated by person-to-person spread through coughing of infected droplets. Plague is a seasonal disease in most countries, occurring during warm and humid times of the year.

The incidence of human plague in 1975, as reported by the World Health Organization, was 1,478 cases with 99 fatalities. In the United States there were 20 cases with four deaths. The following countries reported human plague between 1970 and 1975: in Africa (Angola, Lesotho, Libya, Madagascar, Namibia, Rhodesia, Tanzania, and Zaire); in the Americas (Bolivia, Brazil, Ecuador, Peru), and the United States—Arizona, California, Colorado, New Mexico, and Utah—and in Asia (Burma, Indonesia, and Vietnam) [2].

Pathogenesis

After inoculation of *Y. pestis* into the skin, the bacteria travel via the lymphatics to the regional lymph nodes and are phagocytosed by mononuclear phagocytes, inside which they multiply and develop capsular envelopes [3]. After the incubation period, which is usually two to eight days, the bacteria cause an acute inflammatory response in the lymph node. They are resistant to polymorphonuclear phagocytosis because of their capsules. In the enlarged lymph nodes (buboes), lymphatic obstruction produces local lymphedema, and thrombosis of blood vessels produces hemorrhagic necrosis. The bacteria, which are present in the buboes in massive numbers, intermittently gain access to the bloodstream. Hematogenous dissemination may result in secondary pneumonia or meningitis. Bacteremia with concentrations of $>10^6$ bacteria/ml occasionally occurs with bacilli visible in peripheral blood smears. Under these conditions fatal endotoxemic shock may ensue [4].

Clinical Syndromes

Bubonic plague is the most common clinical form of *Y. pestis* infection. Typically, there is the sudden onset of fever and chills with headache and prostration. The development of the bubo is heralded by painful swelling in the femoral, inguinal, axillary, or cervical region. The onset of fever and the bubo are usually simultaneous, but occasionally the bubo is noticed hours or even days after the initial fever and constitutional symptoms. The pain of the bubo is so excruciating that patients assiduously avoid motion of the affected area and often refuse to allow palpation. Most patients have a single bubo, which is commonly located in the femoral area, but some patients may have them in multiple sites. The buboes are oval swellings about 1–10 cm in length, and may be associated with erythema of the overlying skin [5]. A minority of patients have a pustule or eschar on the area of skin drained by the involved lymph nodes. Palpation of the bubo reveals exquisite tenderness over an unfixed, nonfluctuant mass. Surrounding edema often makes it impossible to distinguish the boundary of the original lymph node from a cluster of matted nodes.

Less common clinical presentations of plague include the septicemic, pneumonic, and meningeal forms. Septicemic plague is a rare variant in which there is no obvious bubo while bacteria are in the bloodstream. Primary pneumonic plague is an inhalation pneumonia resulting from person-to-person transmission. It presents as cough productive of purulent or bloody sputum and can be highly contagious and rapidly fatal. Meningeal plague is rare and usually occurs a week or more after inadequately treated bubonic plague. It results from hematogenous spread from a bubo located commonly in the axilla [4].

Diagnosis

The progression to the diagnosis of plague is shown in figure 1. It should be suspected in febrile patients who have been exposed to rodents or other mammals in the southwestern United States or in other endemic areas of the world. A bacteriologic diagnosis is readily made in most patients by smear and culture of a bubo aspirate. The aspirate is obtained by inserting a 20-gauge needle on a 10-ml syringe containing 1 ml of sterile saline into the bubo and withdrawing several times until the saline becomes blood-tinged. Because the bubo does not contain liquid pus, it may be necessary to inject some of the saline and immediately reaspirate it. Drops of the aspirate should be placed onto microscope slides and air-dried for both Gram and Wayson's stains. The Gram stain will reveal

polymorphonuclear leukocytes and Gram-negative coccobacilli and bacilli ranging from 1 to 2 μm in length. Wayson's stain is prepared by mixing 0.2 g of basic fuchsin (90% dye content) with 0.75 g of methylene blue (90% dye content) in 20 ml of 95% ethyl alcohol. This mixture is then poured slowly into 200 ml of 5% phenol. A smear, after being fixed for 2 min in absolute methanol, is stained for 10–20 sec in Wayson's stain, washed with water, and dried. *Y. pestis* appears as light blue bacilli with dark blue polar bodies, and the remainder of the slide has a contrasting pink counterstain [6]. Smears of blood, sputum, or spinal fluid can be handled similarly.

The aspirate, blood, and other appropriate fluids should be inoculated onto blood and MacConkey's agar plates and into infusion broth. The organism is identified in triple sugar-iron agar by an alkaline slant and acid butt without gas or H_2S, by negative urease and indole reactions, by failure to utilize citrate, and by nonmotility [6]. For definitive identification, cultures should be mailed in double containers to the Center for Disease Control, Plague Branch, P.O. Box 2087, Fort Collins, Colo. 80522 (telephone no., 303–482–0213). At this same laboratory, a serological test, the passive HA test utilizing Fraction I of *Y. pestis,* can be performed on acute- and convalescent-phase serum. In patients with negative cultures, a fourfold or greater increase in titer or a single titer of $\geq$1:16 is presumptive evidence for plague infection.

Management

In 1948 streptomycin was shown to be the drug of choice for the treatment of plague by reducing mortality to <5%. Streptomycin should be administered im in two divided doses totalling 30 mg/kg per day for 10 days [6]. For patients with hypotension requiring iv antibiotics or with meningitis, chloramphenicol should be administered in a loading dose of 25 mg/kg iv followed by 60 mg/kg per day in four divided doses. After clinical improvement, chloramphenicol can be continued orally in the same dose to complete a total course of 10 days.

With successful therapy patients become afebrile in about three days. Although the buboes usually recede without need of local therapy, they occasionally enlarge or become fluctuant during the first week of treatment, requiring incision and drainage. Patients with successfully treated plague almost never have clinical relapses.

All patients with suspected plague must be reported

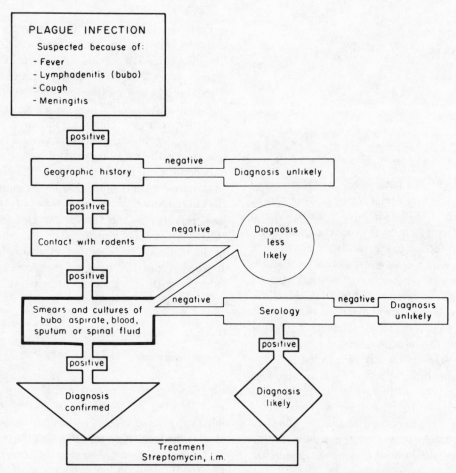

Figure 1. The progression to the diagnosis and management of plague.

to the local health department. Patients with uncomplicated bubonic plague who are promptly treated present little or no health hazard to other persons. Those with cough or other signs of pneumonia, however, must be strictly isolated to prevent airborne spread to other persons. The bubo aspirate and blood must be handled carefully with gloves. Laboratory workers who process the cultures should be alerted to exercise precautions.

A formalin-killed vaccine, Plague Vaccine U.S.P. (Cutter Laboratories, Berkeley, Calif.), is available for travelers to endemic areas who must live and work in close contact with rodents. A primary series of two injections is recommended with a one- to three-month interval between them. Booster injections are given every six months for as long as exposure continues.

References

1. Reed, W. P., Palmer, D. L., Williams, R. C., Kisch, A. L. Bubonic plague in the southwestern United States. Medicine (Balt.)49:465–486, 1970.
2. Human plague in 1975. Wkly. Epidem. Rec. 51:237–239, 1976.
3. Cavanaugh, D. C., Randall, R. The role of multiplication of *Pasturella pestis* in mononuclear phagocytes in the pathogenesis of flea-borne plague. J. Immunol. 83:348–363, 1959.
4. Butler, T., Levin, J., Linh, N. N., Chau, D. M., Adickman, M., Arnold, K. *Yersinia pestis* infection in Vietnam. II. Quantitative blood cultures and detection of endotoxin in the cerebrospinal fluid of patients with meningitis. J. Infect. Dis. 133:493–499, 1976.
5. Butler, T. A clinical study of bubonic plague. Observations of the 1970 Vietnam epidemic with emphasis on coagulation studies, skin histology, and electrocardiograms. Am. J. Med. 53:268–276, 1972.
6. Sonnenwirth, A. C. Yersinia. *In* E. H. Lennette, E. H. Spaulding, and J. P. Truant [ed.]. Manual of clinical microbiology. 2nd ed. American Society for Microbiology, Washington, D.C., 1974, p. 222–225.
7. Meyer, K. F. Modern therapy of plague. J.A.M.A. 144: 982–985, 1950.

Shigellosis

Shigellosis is an acute enteric infection of man caused by the four bacterial species *Shigella dysenteriae, Shigella flexneri, Shigella boydii,* and *Shigella sonnei.* Bacillary dysentery is synonymous with shigellosis. The infection has a worldwide distribution and is prevalent in places where sanitary standards and levels of personal hygiene are low. In the United States, as well as in developing countries, shigellosis persists as a leading cause of diarrheal outbreaks in communities. Man is the major reservoir of shigellae in nature, and the infection is transmitted by the fecal-oral route, often by way of infected hands or fomites, and sometimes by way of contaminated food or water. Clinically, the disease is characterized by abdominal cramps, diarrhea, fever, and stools containing blood and mucus. Although the illness is self-limited with almost negligible mortality, antibiotics can shorten the duration of symptoms and hasten elimination of shigellae from stools.

Epidemiology

Shigella species belong to the family Enterobacteriaceae. They are aerobic, nonmotile, Gram-negative bacilli that are antigenically classified as groups and species [1]. The most common species in the United States is *S. sonnei. S. flexneri* is less common, and *S. boydii* is rare. *S. dysenteriae* type 1 (the Shiga bacillus) is not endemic in the United States but has been imported in travelers.

Man is the major reservoir of infection, as there are no natural animal hosts. During clinical illness and for several days following recovery, organisms are excreted in the stools and may be transmitted to other persons. Infection most often occurs by close person-to-person contact involving contaminated hands, foods, and fomites. Although the organisms may live for prolonged periods in food and water, they do not survive long after drying. There is no evidence for a chronic carrier state, as occurs in typhoid fever.

Persons at highest risk of developing shigellosis are children between the ages of one and four years. Shigellosis usually occurs as outbreaks involving several persons in close contact with one another. These outbreaks are often seen in populations with low hygienic standards, such as institutions for mentally retarded children, Indian reservations, prisons, and military field groups. Travelers to countries with unsanitary restaurants are also at risk of becoming infected [2].

Despite the generally high standards of hygiene in the United States, there were 16,584 cases of shigellosis reported to the Center for Disease Control (CDC, Atlanta, Ga.) in 1975. The monthly incidence in the United States revealed no seasonal variation. In tropical countries, however, there may be seasonal variation with a peak incidence during rainy seasons and when flies are most numerous.

Disease Syndromes

Shigellae are efficient pathogens in man as demonstrated by the fact that as few as 200 ingested bacilli initiated disease in 25% of healthy volunteers [3]. During the incubation period, which is usually 36–72 hr, the organisms traverse the small bowel and proliferate. Enterotoxin-induced secretion of fluid in the small bowel explains the watery diarrhea that occurs early in the illness [4]. In the colon *Shigellae* attain concentrations of 10^6–10^{10} organisms/g of stool. The bacilli possess invasive capabilities, allowing them to penetrate the colonic epithelium. The bacteria multiply further within epithelial cells leading to an acute inflammatory response with resultant mucosal ulceration, distortion of villus architecture, and formation of microabscesses. Long segments of colon may be affected with diffuse colitis. The mucosa is friable and covered with an exudate of polymorphonuclear leukocytes. Consequently, the stool often contains red blood cells and polymorphonuclear leukocytes. Bacteremia occurs only occasionally, and colonic perforation is not a complication of this superficial inflammatory process. Although the mortality rate of shigellosis is <1% in the United States, death may result, especially in young children, from excessive loss of fluid.

Initial symptoms are usually cramping abdominal pain and fever accompanied by watery diarrhea and tenesmus. Dysentery (passage of blood and mucus), when present, usually appears a day or more after the onset of the disease. In this later stage of the illness, fever may be absent so that some patients will present with afebrile, bloody diarrhea. In children the fever may reach high levels. Nausea and vomiting may occur at any stage of the illness. Abdominal examination often shows lower quadrant abdominal tenderness and hyperactive bowel sounds. It should be noted that shigellosis produces a spectrum of clinical disease from mild symptoms with minimal amounts of watery diarrhea to severe toxicity with grossly bloody stools.

Diagnosis

Figure 1 shows the progression to the diagnosis and management of shigellosis. Infection with *Shigella* should be suspected in anyone with diarrhea, with or without fever. The diagnosis is more likely, however, in high-risk groups such as children, persons living in institutions with low sanitary standards, and travelers recently returned from areas with substandard sanitary conditions. Examination for leukocytes should be performed with a portion of liquid stool, preferably containing blood or mucus. A fleck or drop of stool is placed on a microscope slide and mixed thoroughly with two drops of methylene blue solution (0.3 g of methylene blue dissolved in 30 ml of ethyl alcohol, added to 100 ml of 0.01% potassium hydroxide solution). A cover slip is placed over the mixture of stool and methylene blue solution, and the slide is examined under the microscope through the high-power ob-

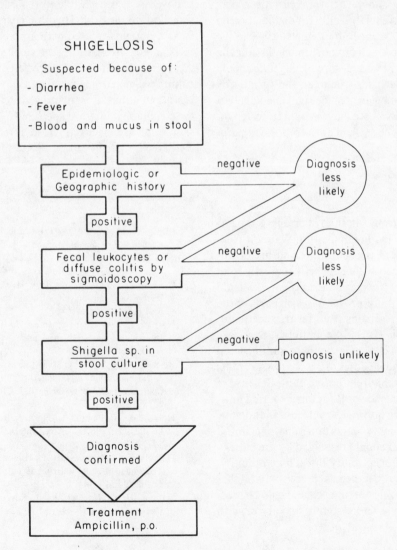

Figure 1.   The progression to a diagnosis and treatment of shigellosis; p.o. = perorally.

jective. In shigellosis polymorphonuclear leukocytes are usually abundant [5], but this finding is not diagnostic. Sigmoidoscopic examination of the colon in shigellosis often reveals diffuse erythema and friability of the mucosa. Ulcers, if present, are usually shallow and 3–7 mm in diameter.

Freshly passed stool or mucosal swabs obtained at the time of sigmoidoscopy should be promptly cultured. If a delay of more than a few hours is anticipated in culturing a specimen of stool, the stool should be placed in a buffered glycerol-saline solution for preservation. This solution can be prepared by combining 4.2 g of NaCl, 3.1 g of anhydrous dipotassium phosphate, 1.0 g of anhydrous monopotassium phosphate, 0.003 g of phenol red, 700 ml of distilled water, and 300 ml of glycerol [1].

Stool specimens should be streaked onto blood, xylose-lysine-deoxycholate, and salmonella-shigella agars. All species except *S. dysenteriae* type 1 (the Shiga bacillus) grow well on the salmonella-shigella agar. Selected colonies suggestive of shigellae should be placed on triple sugar-iron agar and lysine-iron agar. Colonies showing an alkaline slant and acid butt without gas or H_2S in both agars should be tested for agglutination with polyvalent antisera for *Shigella*.

Management

Antibiotics are effective both in shortening the duration of diarrhea and in eliminating *Shigella* from stools [6]. Because of the self-limited nature of shigellosis, some patients will not benefit clinically from antibiotic therapy. Nevertheless, antibiotics should be given to most culture-proven cases, in part for the protection of other persons from fecal excretion of shigellae. Ampicillin (Bristol Laboratories, Syracuse, N.Y.) is the drug of choice. It should be administered orally in four individual doses of 2 g per day to adults and 100 mg/kg to children for five days. Because of the increasing frequency of R factor-mediated antimicrobial resistance in *Shigella* infections, antibiotic susceptibility testing is important, and the initial choice of antibiotics should be guided by the pattern of antimicrobial susceptibility in each community. When ampicillin resistance is present, trimethoprim-sulfamethoxazole or tetracycline should be used. In rare cases with severe systemic toxicity or with

profuse colonic bleeding, there is an indication for antibiotics before results of the stool cultures are available.

In addition to antibiotics, rehydration with intravenous fluids will be required by patients who have lost an excessive volume of diarrhea fluid. Ringer's lactate is a good choice for isotonic volume replacement. Rarely, blood loss in the stool will be great enough to require blood transfusions. The commonly used drug for reduction of intestinal motility, Lomotil® (Searle Laboratories, Chicago, Ill.), may prolong the duration of diarrhea and excretion of *Shigella* and should, therefore, be avoided [7].

For the protection of families and other contacts, patients should be advised to practice particularly careful hand washing following defecation for at least two weeks. It is desirable to report all patients with shigellosis to the State Health Department. Although 92% of patients treated with ampicillin were shown to have negative cultures of stool specimens by 10 days after initiation of therapy [6], a follow-up stool culture will determine whether a convalescent patient is still infectious. For the prevention of shigellosis in the community, improved personal hygiene and public sanitation are necessary. No effective vaccine is available for general use.

References

1. Ewing, W. H., Martin, W. J. Enterobacteriaceae. *In* E. H. Lennette, E. H. Spaulding, and J. P. Truant [ed.]. Manual of clinical microbiology. 2nd ed. American Society for Microbiology, Washington, D.C., 1974. p. 189–213, 896.
2. Gangarosa, E. J. Shigellosis. *In* F. H. Top and P. F. Wehrle [ed.]. Communicable and infectious diseases. C. V. Mosby, St. Louis, 1976. p. 616–622.
3. Hornick, R. B. Bacillary dysentery. *In* P. D. Hoeprich [ed.]. Infectious diseases. Harper and Row, Hagerstown, 1972, p. 603–609.
4. Keusch, G. T., Grady, G. F., Mata, L. J., McIver, J. The pathogenesis of *Shigella* diarrhea. I. Enterotoxin production by *Shigella dysenteriae* I. J. Clin. Invest. 51:1212–1218, 1972.
5. Harris, J. C., DuPont, H. L., Hornick, R. B. Fecal leukocytes in diarrheal illness. Ann. Intern. Med. 76:697–703, 1972.
6. Haltalin, K. C., Kusmiesz, H. T., Hinton, L. V., Nelson, J. D. Treatment of acute diarrhea in outpatients. Am. J. Dis. Child. 124:554–561, 1972.
7. DuPont, H. L., Hornick, R. B. Adverse effect of lomotil therapy in shigellosis. J.A.M.A. 226:1525–1528, 1973.

Tuberculosis

Throughout most of history tuberculosis has been a major and common disease of man. Viewed globally today, it may be the most important specifically identifiable and readily treatable human disease. One-half of the population of the world is infected with *Mycobacterium tuberculosis,* and tuberculosis is the most common cause of death among reported infections. Most parts of Latin America, Africa, India, Southeast Asia and Southern Asia have high case rates of tuberculosis. For example, recent rates of infection in many Latin American countries are two to eight times higher than those in the United States, and these figures are minimal estimates because of underreporting in many countries.

In the United States, the incidence of tuberculosis and related deaths has been declining steadily during the past century, for which data are available. Today most Americans reach adulthood uninfected. The cases of tuberculosis that do occur tend to cluster in identifiable, high-risk segments of the population. Additional risk is imposed upon Americans today because of the increased frequency of travel to areas of high prevalence of tuberculosis. Ochs reported the development of tuberculosis on a U.S. Navy ship stationed in the Mediterranean [1]. One member of the crew contracted tuberculosis after intimate contact with an infected local civilian. Subsequently, three additional cases of tuberculosis and 58 infections without disease developed in the 236 personnel aboard the ship who were in contact with the index case. The transmission of tuberculosis to American civilians by military personnel who have returned from overseas service has also been documented.

Today many American medical students complete their education without ever seeing a case of tuberculosis, and many of these students will pursue the four decades of their professional careers without treating a patient with tuberculosis. Concomitantly with this decrease in tuberculosis, the skilled cadre of physicians trained in treatment of tuberculosis that was spawned by the sanitorium movement of the prechemotherapy era is disappearing, and the re-sponsibility for treatment and prevention of this disease is being turned over to the general community of the medical profession.

The majority of cases of tuberculosis in the United States today occur in elderly individuals and are the legacy of previously high rates of infection. Other cases occur in younger, recently infected individuals. Some such infections are sporadic, but many can be traced to contacts or occur in microepidemics. The diagnosis is frequently missed or made after inappropriate delay in general health facilities where personnel have little experience with this disease. Special problems are created by the very long interval which often separates infection and disease, by unwarranted concern over infectiousness, and by social stigmatization of tuberculosis patients.

Epidemiology

Tuberculosis results from infection with *M. tuberculosis.* This infection almost always results from person-to-person transmission via the aerial route. The control of bovine tuberculosis in all countries where there is significant milk consumption has all but eliminated this orally acquired form of tuberculosis. Not all patients with tuberculosis are contagious, and not all environments are equally conducive to the transmission of *M. tuberculosis.* Within a contaminated environment, the risk of being infected is solely determined by the statistical probability of inhaling airborne organisms, but the risk of subsequent disease is highly variable and depends on many host factors.

Cough, extensive pulmonary disease (particularly with cavitation), and large numbers of bacilli in expectorated sputum distinguish those persons with tuberculosis who are most infectious. After initiation of drug therapy, patients become noninfectious rapidly, usually within two weeks. The great majority of infectious patients actually discharge relatively few organisms, and the risk of casual or brief contact with these patients is negligible. Tubercle bacilli remain suspended in air for a long time, and ventilation is the most important environmental factor influencing transmission. Closed rooms provide very favorable circumstances for the spread of tuberculosis, whereas there is virtually no risk of spread outdoors. Nonrecirculating air-conditioning systems greatly decrease the risk of infection, and the high turnover rate of air in American hospitals makes elaborate isolation procedures unnecessary. Residual dust fomites are not a source of infection. From these considerations it is easy to understand that most transmission of tuberculous infection occurs in the home and that the risk of household contacts ceases promptly with treatment of the index case. It is also evident that under conditions of high prevalence of tuberculosis most infections are acquired early in life from parents or grandparents.

The risk to uninfected American tourists traveling overseas in areas of high prevalence of tuberculosis is negligible. Even Americans residing in areas where tuberculosis occurs frequently are at little risk, unless they live in the home of a contagious patient or unless such a patient is living in their home. Tuberculous servants may present a particular hazard to American children abroad. Of more serious concern to American physicians are those individuals immigrating to the United States from regions where tuberculosis is highly prevalent. Many such persons will have been infected prior to arrival in the United States. Among 59,309 Vietnamese refugees screened after entrance into the United States in 1975, 2,031 (3.4%) had X-ray findings that suggested tuberculosis, and 264 persons were found with samples of sputum positive for *M. tuberculosis* [2]. Of tuberculin tests in children 14 years old or younger, 12.4% were positive.

Among persons who become infected with tubercle bacilli, disease occurs in only about 5%. The disease occurs mostly within the first few years of infection, except that school-age children tend to defer their illness until the postpubertal years of young adulthood. However, many decades of healthy life may separate infection in childhood from disease in the senescent years. Most infected individuals have sufficient immunity so that exogenous reinfection does not occur, and clinical disease, even in persons many years past their primary infections, represents reactivation of previously acquired infection.

At present in the United States, three of four cases of tuberculosis occur in the elderly. The classical cohort analysis of Frost [3] demonstrated that these patients represent the remaining legacy of an earlier time when most Americans were exposed to great risk of infection in childhood. Today 97% of Americans reach adulthood uninfected [4].

For the most part, the factors that predispose individuals to the development of tuberculosis are unknown. Among known factors alcoholism, corticosteroid and immunosuppressive therapy, malnutrition, cachexia from wasting diseases, defective cellular hypersensitivity, silicosis, and labile diabetes can be listed. Moreover, most tuberculosis in the United States today occurs in economically poor, highly urban areas. These factors, in addition to older age and a history of contact at any age with tuberculous household members, designate those persons in whom American physicians should most suspect tuberculosis.

Disease Syndromes

Most tuberculous patients present with pulmonary disease. The clinician should particularly suspect this disease in patients with chronic pneumonitis, especially of the upper lobes, when signs of acute sepsis are not prominent. Cavitation strongly suggests tuberculosis. Many tuberculosis patients are asymptomatic. Cough and weight loss are the most common complaints, and drenching night sweats involving the upper half of the body are characteristic. Fever is usually low-grade.

Extrapulmonary tuberculosis is less common, and signs and symptoms are referable to the site of involvement. Common sites of involvement are cervical lymph nodes, the thoracic spine and paraspinous psoas space, meninges and brain, kidneys, epididymis and Fallopian tubes, pleura and peritoneum, and synovial membranes. Any tissue or organ in the body may be involved. Miliary tuberculosis should always be considered in the differential diagnosis of fever of unknown origin, even in the presence of a normal chest X ray and negative tuberculin test.

Diagnosis

The accompanying algorithm (figure 1) outlines a logical approach to diagnosis. Tuberculous infection is usually suspected either because of a clinical illness consistent with tuberculosis or because of an epidemiologic history that suggests exposure to persons with infectious tuberculosis. The tuberculin skin test is the primary tool available for the recognition of individuals infected with *M. tuberculosis* [5]. Of such persons, 95% will react to a properly performed test. The standard procedure is an intradermal injection of 5 test units (0.0001 mg) of tuberculin purified protein derivative (PPD). When tuberculosis remains suspected clinically in the presence of a negative result

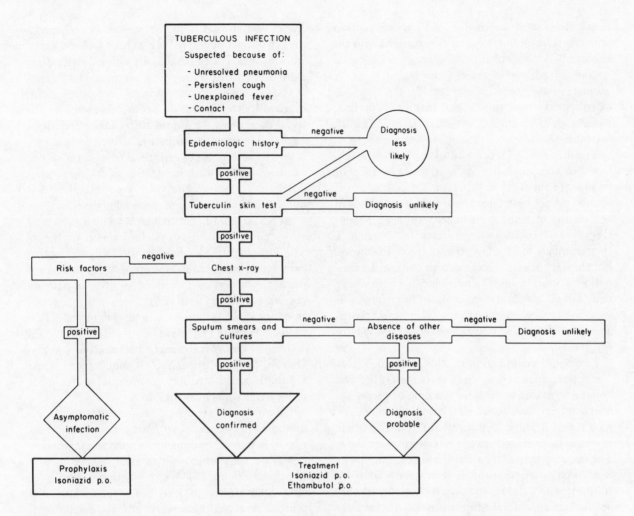

Figure 1.   Progression to logical evaluation and management of infection with Mycobacterium tuberculosis.

with the PPD test, the test should be repeated in a few days; a 5 test unit-dose should once again be used. Weak reactivity is often boosted by the first test so that the patient is readily recognized as a positive reactor upon retesting.

Interpretation of tuberculin test reactions requires considerable care. The size of the reaction must be known accurately in terms of the mean diameter in millimeters of induration at 48–72 hr. Standards for the interpretation of PPD reactions are given in table 1. The published statement of the American Thoracic Society Committee on Diagnostic Skin Testing [6][1] is a useful guide.

Once the presence of infection with *M. tuberculosis*

has been established, the question of whether or not the patient has disease may be addressed. Most tuberculosis is pulmonary, and the chest X ray is of major diagnostic importance. Review of prior X rays

Table 1.   Interpretation of reactions to skin tests performed with 5 test units of tuberculin purified protein derivative given intradermally.

Diameter of reaction at 48–72 hr (mm)	Interpretation
0–4	Negative. Patient probably not infected with *Mycobacterium tuberculosis*
5–9	Equivocal. Hypersensitivity may be due to *Mycobacterium* other than *M. tuberculosis*
≥10	Positive. Patient probably infected with *M. tuberculosis*

[1] Reprints of current revisions of statements from the American Thoracic Society are available from local offices of the American Lung Association.

is usually helpful, and one should never accept an opinion that a pulmonary lesion consistent with tuberculosis is inactive, unless this judgment is based on the comparison of remote and recent films. A normal chest X ray essentially excludes the diagnosis of pulmonary tuberculosis, and further evaluation, including examination of sputum, then becomes unwarranted.

The diagnosis of tuberculosis is ultimately established by the demonstration of tubercle bacilli. For pulmonary tuberculosis, sputum is examined, or if sputum cannot be obtained, gastric aspirate obtained in the early morning is examined. Although nonpathogenic mycobacteria may be present in the stomach, their numbers are too few to be detected in smears, but they are readily recognized in culture. Examination of sputum should always include both smear and culture. Duplicate smears from two samples of sputum have a yield equal to one culture, and the diagnostic information is available more rapidly with smears.

Kinyoun's modification of the classical Ziehl-Neelsen technique [7] is excellent for most office and hospital ward use; reagents for this staining procedure are commercially available (TB stain kit K, catalogue no. 3326-32-3; Difco, Detroit, Mich.). A thick particle of sputum is crushed between two microscopic slides and smeared by pulling apart the slides. The smear is allowed to air dry and is then gently fixed by warming with a flame. The slide is covered with carbol fuchsin stain for 3 min, rinsed, decolorized exhaustively with 3% concentrated HCl in 95% ethyl alcohol, and counterstained for 1 min with brilliant green stain. The stained smear must be examined with an oil immersion lens, and careful examination for several minutes is often required to find the brilliant red, slender, curved tubercle bacilli. If smears are negative, cultures should always be performed on several specimens. Occasionally, biopsy is required for the diagnosis of tuberculosis, especially when lymph nodes are involved. Biopsy specimens should always be cultured in addition to being submitted for histologic examination.

Management

The initial treatment of tuberculosis for almost all adult patients in the United States should consist of 300 mg of isoniazid (Ciba Pharmaceutical Co., Summit, N.J.; Kasar Laboratories, Niles, Ill,; Eli Lilly and Company, Indianapolis, Ind.; Nydrazide,®

E. R. Squibb and Sons, Princeton, N.J.) and 15 mg/kg of ethambutol (Myambutol,® Lederle Laboratories, Pearl River, N.Y.) in a single daily dose. Both drugs are extremely well tolerated, and toxicity is infrequently encountered. Allergic reactions, especially drug fevers, occur uncommonly. At the usual dose there is no need to be concerned about isoniazid-induced neuropathy, except in patients otherwise susceptible to peripheral neuropathy, which can be avoided by administration of 50 mg of pyridoxine daily. Optic neuropathy due to ethambutol is not a problem with the recommended dose.

Isoniazid drug hepatitis has become a subject of major concern among physicians treating patients with tuberculosis [8]. Clinically it is indistinguishable from viral hepatitis and often progresses to death if use of the drug is continued. Monitoring of patients receiving isoniazid with serial serum enzyme determination is not helpful. p-Aminosalicylic acid (Pascorbic,® Hellwig Pharmaceuticals, Chicago, Ill.; Eli Lilly and Company; Pamisyl,® Parke, Davis and Co., Detroit, Mich.; Rezipas,® E. R. Squibb and Sons) should be substituted for ethambutol for treatment of pregnant women and children.

Uninterrupted treatment must be continued for a minimum of one year; two years is a more usual period of therapy. The outcome of such treatment is so favorable, with subsequent rates of relapse of <1% [9], that continued follow-up study is unnecessary for adequately treated patients. Rest, special diet, and other general health measures add nothing to treatment when adequate chemotherapy is given [10] and may divert resources which are better expended on assuring continued, uninterrupted therapy.

Retreatment after relapse or failure of initial treatment always presents a difficult problem and usually requires consultation with an experienced specialist. In vitro drug susceptibility tests of the organisms isolated from the patient are necessary. When rifampin (Rimactane,® Ciba Pharmaceutical Co.; Rifadin,® Dow Pharmaceuticals, Indianapolis, Ind.) has not been previously used, administration of rifampin and one other new drug may be started, pending results of susceptibility tests. If rifampin has been used initially, then four new drugs are commonly required for retreatment. Therapy with isoniazid should usually be continued.

It is not sufficient to limit concern to those patients with tuberculous disease. The elegant clinical trials of the U.S. Public Health Service [11] have demonstrated that isoniazid prophylaxis can be of great benefit to those who are infected but free of disease.

With confidence limits of 95%, such infected individuals can be recognized by results of tuberculin tests [5].

The selection of persons for isoniazid prophylaxis depends largely on the consideration of potential benefit as balanced against the potential risk of isoniazid drug hepatitis [8]. The guidelines of the American Thoracic Society [12] are well drawn and extremely helpful in this regard. In general, persons considered for isoniazid prophylaxis should include all those younger than 35 years with positive PPD reactions, all close household contacts of untreated, infectious patients with tuberculosis, all persons with clearly documented, recent conversions in PPD skin tests, and all PPD-positive individuals older than 35 years with special risk factors favoring the development of pulmonary diseases. The proper therapeutic regimen is 300 mg of isoniazid daily in a single dose for one year.

It must always be remembered that tuberculosis is an infectious disease which must be reported to the local health department. The investigation of family contacts, who are often candidates for isoniazid prophylaxis, is usually carried out by local health department personnel.

References

1. Ochs, C. W. The epidemiology of tuberculosis. J.A.M.A. 179:247–252, 1962.

2. Center for Disease Control. Update on Vietnamese refugee health status. Morbidity and Mortality Weekly Rep. 24: 267–268, 1975.

3. Frost, W. H. The age selection of mortality from tuberculosis in successive decades. Am. J. Hyg. 30:91–96, 1939.

4. Edwards, L. B., Acquaviva, F. A., Livesay, V. T., Cross, F. W., Palmer, C. E. An atlas of sensitivity to tuberculin, PPD-B, and histoplasmin in the United States. Am. Rev. Resp. Dis. 99(Suppl.):1–132, 1969.

5. Edwards, P. Q., Edwards, L. B. Story of the tuberculin test from an epidemiologic viewpoint. Am. Rev. Resp. Dis. 81(Suppl.):1–47, 1960.

6. American Thoracic Society Committee on Diagnostic Skin Testing. The tuberculin skin test. Am. Rev. Resp. Dis. 104:769–775, 1971.

7. Bailey, R. W., Scott, E. G. Diagnostic microbiology. C. V. Mosby Co., St. Louis, Mo., 1974, p. 389.

8. Mitchell, J. R., Zimmerman, H. J., Ishak, K. G., Thorgeirsson, U. P., Timbrell, J. A., Snodgrass, W. R., Nelson, S. D. Isoniazid liver injury: clinical spectrum, pathology, and probable pathogenesis. Ann. Intern. Med. 84:181–192, 1976.

9. Stead, W. W., Jurgens, G. H. Productivity of prolonged follow-up after chemotherapy for tuberculosis. Am. Rev. Resp. Dis. 108:314–320, 1973.

10. Dawson, J. J. Y., Devadatta, S., Fox, W., Radhakrishna, S., Ramakrishnan, C. V., Somasundaram, P. R., Stott, H., Tripathy, S. P., Velu, S. A 5-year study of patients with pulmonary tuberculosis in a concurrent comparison of home and sanatorium treatment for one year with isoniazid plus PAS. Bull. W.H.O. 34:533–551, 1966.

11. Ferebee, S. H. Controlled chemoprophylaxis trials in tuberculosis. A general review. Adv. Tuberc. Res. 17:28–106, 1970.

12. American Thoracic Society. Preventive therapy of tuberculous infection. Am. Rev. Resp. Dis. 110:371–374, 1974.

Typhoid Fever

Typhoid fever is a bacterial infection of man caused by *Salmonella typhi*. The organism is transmitted by the fecal-oral route via contaminated water and food. Although present throughout the world, *S. typhi* infection is particularly prevalent in countries with warm climates and with less developed sanitary facilities for sewage disposal and water treatment. Nevertheless, several hundred cases are diagnosed annually in the United States. Clinically, typhoid fever is characterized by prolonged fever, abdominal pain, rash, splenomegaly, and hepatomegaly. Although typhoid fever is often included among diarrheal diseases, it is important to note that diarrhea is an uncommon feature of this disease. The mortality rate may be high, and death is related to severe toxemia, intestinal hemorrhage, or intestinal perforation. Treatment with chloramphenicol or other effective drugs shortens the course of fever and significantly reduces mortality.

Epidemiology

Man is the only natural host for *S. typhi*. Persons of all ages and both sexes appear to be equally susceptible to infection. Experimental evidence suggests that alteration of intestinal flora by antibiotics allows infection to develop more readily. The chronic helminthic infection schistosomiasis may predispose persons both to typhoid fever and to a chronic urinary carrier state. The chronic intestinal carrier state more often develops in females and in persons older than 50 years.

Typhoid fever is endemic in most of the countries of Central and South America, Africa, and Asia. In the United States the annual incidence has steadily declined since 1900, but about 400 cases have been reported annually during the last few years. The incubation period, which is usually eight to 14 days, permits travelers to develop typhoid fever after returning from areas where the disease is endemic, such as Mexico. A large proportion of the cases reported in the United States were either in recent travelers to Mexico or in individuals with Hispanic surnames. Furthermore, the case rates for California and Texas are five times higher than those for other states [1]. The monthly incidence of typhoid fever in the United States reveals no seasonal variation.

Man is the only source of infection in nature, as *S. typhi* has no known animal reservoirs or vectors. Patients with symptomatic infections continue to excrete *S. typhi* in both urine and feces even while being treated. About 3% of patients recovering from typhoid fever become chronic carriers who excrete up to 10^{11} bacteria/g of feces continually for years and are important sources of new infection in the community. In addition, *S. typhi* can survive for prolonged periods in water, ice, dust, and dried sewage, which subsequently may become sources of infection.

Clinical Syndromes

Persons become infected by ingesting water or food containing *S. typhi*. The number of bacteria required to initiate disease in 50% of healthy volunteers was found to be 10^7, and the incubation period averaged 7.5 days [2]. Incubation periods may be longer, up to 33 days, with exposure to lower doses of bacteria [2]. The ingested bacilli cross the small intestinal mucosa to enter the lymphatics and are phagocytized in Peyer's patches and regional lymph nodes. During the incubation period bacilli proliferate in mononuclear phagocytes of lymphoid tissue and then gain access to the blood. In the first two weeks of symptomatic disease, there is a sustained bacteremia, and bacilli reach reticuloendothelial cells of the liver, spleen, and bone marrow, where mononuclear cells proliferate. During the second and third weeks of illness, infection of the biliary tract results in increasing numbers of *S. typhi* in the feces. In untreated or progressive disease the lymphoid tissue of Peyer's patches enlarges, leading to necrosis and ulceration of adjacent intestinal mucosa or to intestinal perforation. Patients may die in these later stages of the disease for unknown reasons with a clinical picture of severe toxemia and exhaustion.

There is wide variation in clinical severity. Typically the onset of illness is gradual with mild and remitting symptoms of fever, headache, myalgia, anorexia, and dry cough. Physical signs other than fever are usually absent during the first week of illness. During the second week of illness, the symptoms, including abdominal discomfort, become more sustained and intense, leading to prostration. Most patients have some degree of abdominal tenderness, usually in the lower quadrants, and distention is common. The liver and spleen are commonly palpable and are usually not tender. Constipation is more common than diarrhea. Rose spots, which are small maculopapular erythematous lesions, appear most commonly on the upper abdomen. Melena may be present or bright red blood may be passed through the rectum. If untreated, the disease may progress to sustained high fever with severe lethargy or delirium. Intestinal perforation should be suspected in patients with abdominal rigidity or ileus.

Normochromic anemia develops during the course of illness and may be exacerbated by intestinal blood loss. The white blood cell count is usually normal but may be decreased. Platelet counts are frequently decreased. Liver function tests often reveal moderately increased levels of transaminase and bilirubin.

Diagnosis

An algorithm for the diagnosis and treatment of typhoid fever is shown in figure 1. Typhoid fever should be suspected in persons with fever persisting for longer than a week, especially if they have been in areas where the disease is endemic or have been exposed to known typhoid carriers. A blood culture is the most useful diagnostic test for typhoid fever. Positive blood cultures for *S. typhi* can be obtained in ~90% of patients during the first week of illness and in ~50% of patients after the third week. In these later stages of illness, increasing numbers of stool and urine cultures become positive, and bone marrow cultures are more frequently positive than blood cultures.

S. typhi, a Gram-negative bacillus in the family Enterobacteriaceae, is identified by an alkaline slant and acid butt without gas in triple sugar-iron agar, by failure to grow on Simmons' citrate, by a negative urease reaction, and by serologic testing for somatic and flagellar antigens. Serological tests are not a satisfactory substitute for bacteriological studies. In the absence of recent immunization, however, a fourfold or greater increase in titer of *Salmonella* O agglutinin can be used as confirmatory evidence for the diagnosis.

Management

Chloramphenicol has remained the drug of choice for typhoid fever since its introduction in 1948 [3]. The use of chloramphenicol reduced the mortality rate of typhoid fever from ~12% to ~4% [4]. Most patients become afebrile three to five days after the onset of treatment. Chloramphenicol (Parke-Davis and Co., Detroit, Mich.) is given orally in a dose of 50–60 mg/kg body weight per day, given as 4 equal portions every 6 hr. After defervescence and clinical improvement the dosage can be reduced to 30 mg/kg body weight per day. The duration of therapy should be 14 days. In patients unable to take oral medication, the same dosage should be given im until the patient can take tablets.

Patients who are dehydrated or anorectic or who have diarrhea will require iv saline with attention to possible electrolyte and acid-base disturbances. Patients with brisk intestinal bleeding will require blood transfusion. Therapy for suspected intestinal perforation should be nasogastric suction and the addition of gentamicin (Schering Corp., Bloomfield, N.J.) given im in a dose of 3 mg/kg per day. Surgery should be reserved for patients who develop intestinal obstruction or an abcess following perforation [5].

Alternative drugs to chloramphenicol should be used when infection with *S. typhi* resistant to chloramphenicol is suspected. In 1972 and 1973 in Mexico, India, Vietnam, and Thailand, isolates of *S. typhi* from patients were shown to harbor an episome encoding resistance to chloramphenicol, tetracycline, streptomycin, and sulfonamides [6]. Therefore, patients returning from those or other countries reporting chloramphenicol resistance should be treated initially with ampicillin. Ampicillin (Bristol Laboratories, Syracuse, N.Y.) must be given iv in a dose of 60–80 mg/kg of body weight per day in four equal portions every 6 hr for 14 days. If cultures subsequently reveal *S. typhi* susceptible to chloramphenicol, chloramphenicol should be substituted for ampicillin.

Patients with typhoid fever should have specimens of stools tested regularly for isolation of *S. typhi* and should be reported to the local Health Department. After recovery of patients, stool cultures should be performed once a month until negative. Carriers should be prevented from working as food-handlers. Chronic carriers (persons excreting bacilli more than a year after their illness) should be treated with ampicillin (100 mg/kg of body weight orally in four

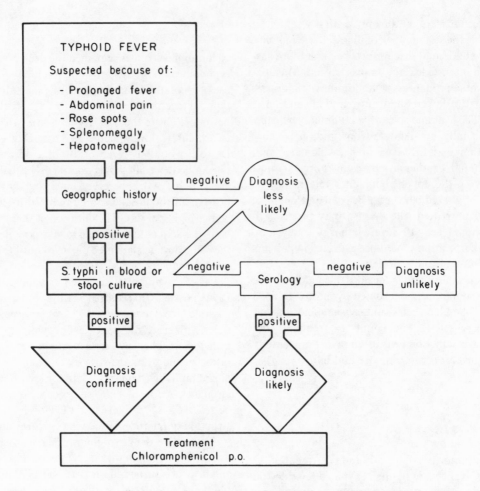

Figure 1.   The progression to the diagnosis and management of typhoid fever due to *Salmonella typhi*;
p.o. = perorally.

equal portions every 6 hr daily) and probenecid
(Merck Sharp and Dohme, West Point, Pa.) (30
mg/kg of body weight per day given as four equal
portions every 6 hr orally) for four to six weeks. Patients with gallstones or evidence of gallbladder disease may require cholecystectomy for eradication of
the carrier state [4].

Prophylaxis

Travelers going to areas where typhoid fever is endemic should be advised concerning vaccination and
avoidance of uncooked foods and unprocessed water.
Although not required by law, typhoid vaccine has
been shown to be moderately effective in field trials.
Typhoid vaccine, U.S.P. (Wyeth Laboratories,
Philadelphia, Pa.), is administered as two sc injections

of 0.5 ml at an interval of about four weeks. A booster
dose is given every three years if needed. The protection provided by the vaccine, which is only partial,
can be overcome by ingestion of large numbers of
bacilli. Therefore, vaccination appears to be a relatively less important preventive measure than dietary
precautions.

References

1. Weissman, J. B., Rice, P. A., Krogstad, D. J., Baine, W. B.,
    Gangarosa, E. J. Risk of severe intestinal infection to the
    traveler in Mexico. J. Infect. Dis. 128:574–578, 1973.
2. Hornick, R. B., Greisman, S. E., Woodward, T. E., DuPont,
    H. L., Dawkins, A. T., Snyder, M. J. Typhoid fever:
    pathogenesis and immunologic control. N. Engl. J. Med.
    283:686–691, 739–746, 1970.
3. Snyder, M. J., Perroni, J., Gonzalez, O., Woodward, W. E.,
    Palomino, C., Gonzalez, C., Music, S. I., DuPont, H. L.,
    Hornick, R. B., Woodward, T. E. Comparative efficacy of

chloramphenicol, ampicillin, and co-trimoxazole in the treatment of typhoid fever. Lancet 2:1155–1157, 1976.

4. Woodward, T. E., Smadel, J. E. Management of typhoid fever and its complications. Ann. Intern. Med. 60:144–157, 1964.

5. Hook, E. W., Johnson, W. D. Typhoid fever. *In* P. D. Hoeprich [ed.]. Infectious diseases. Harper and Row, Hagerstown, Maryland, 1972, p. 599–600.

6. Anderson, E. S., Smith, H. R. Chloramphenicol resistance in the typhoid bacillus. Br. Med. J. 3:329–331, 1972.

Amebiasis

Infection with the protozoan parasite *Entamoeba histolytica* has a cosmopolitan distribution, with the prevalence varying between 5% in temperate areas to 80% in some tropical communities. The primary habitat of *E. histolytica* is the gastro-intestinal tract, where in the majority of cases the protozoa appear to be largely confined to the lumen. Under as yet unknown circumstances, which may involve either host or parasite factors, *E. histolytica* invades the intestinal mucosa, often leading to diarrhea and dysentery. From the intestines the organisms may also pass to other organs, particularly the liver, where they can initiate abscess formation.

In the United States, *E. histolytica* infection was first described as a cause of dysentery by Osler in 1890 [1]. Overall estimates of the prevalence of infection vary between 3% and 10%; this wide variation is due to difficulty in differentiation of *E. histolytica* from other closely related organisms. With the recent enormous increase in worldwide travel, more imported infections are being reported in this country. The risk of contracting amebiasis abroad is illustrated by the observation that, of 667 Peace Corps volunteers who were stationed in India, 57% were infected and 17% had invasive disease [2].

Life Cycle

The life cycle of *E. histolytica* involves a spectrum of morphological stages, with the active trophozoites at one pole and the resistant cysts at the other. The commensal trophozoites of *E. histolytica* live and multiply in the lumen of the large intestine, especially the cecum. These forms measure 10–20 μm in diameter with a nucleus that contains a small central karyosome and fine granular peripheral chromatin. As the contents of the large bowel advance and become less fluid, the trophozoites change into round or oval cysts, which at maturity measure 10–18 μm in diameter and contain four nuclei. The cysts, which are resistant to the external environment, are passed in the feces. On ingestion by a susceptible host, the cyst wall is destroyed in the gastrointestinal tract, the nuclei double in number, and eight trophozoites are released. In invasive, clinically apparent amebiasis, the trophozoites enlarge to as much as 50 μm in diameter and ingest red blood cells which may be seen within vacuoles in the cytoplasm.

Epidemiology

Man is the reservoir of *E. histolytica* and passes the infection to other primates, cats, dogs, and, rarely, pigs. Amebiasis spreads by ingestion of cysts since trophozoites are rapidly destroyed by both external environmental conditions and gastric acidity. Cysts, on the other hand, may survive in soil for at least eight days at 28 C–34 C, for 40 days at 2 C–6 C, and for 62 days at 0 C. Although cysts are not affected by the concentration of chlorine usually present in water purification procedures, they are removed by the sand filtration step. Cysts are destroyed by 200 ppm of iodine, 5%–10% acetic acid, or boiling.

Amebiasis is transmitted by food and drink contaminated with cysts. Food handlers harboring amebic cysts seem to play the most important role in transmission. Raw vegetables and fruit that are washed in polluted water and food exposed to filth flies are also sources of infection.

Of the three species of *Entamoeba* that commonly infect man (*coli, hartmanni,* and *histolytica*), only *E. histolytica* has been shown to be pathogenic. The larger *E. coli* and the similar, but smaller, *E. hartmanni* (formerly called the small race of *E. histolytica*; cysts <10 μm in diameter) are both nonpathogenic.

Clinical Syndromes

After infection of the human host with *E. histolytica,* the amebae usually remain within the bowel lumen as commensals. Gross invasion of the host tissues occurs only in a small proportion of individuals (2%–8%). The invasiveness of *E. histolytica* has been said to be related to a variety of factors, including the strain of the parasite and the nutritional status and intestinal bacterial flora of the host, but these relations have not been conclusively established. The greater pathogenicity of amebiasis in certain locations, such as South Africa and Mexico, also remains to be explained. The most common presentations of disease due to *E. histolytica* are related to local invasion of the gut mucosa or dissemination of the organisms to other organs, particularly the liver [3].

(1) Intestinal amebiasis. As illustrated in one large series of cases, in 71% of patients the onset of intestinal disease was gradual with abdominal pain that was often colicky in nature and with frequent bowel movements; tenesmus occurred in 91% of cases [3]. With the establishment of dysentery, the number of bowel movements, which contained variable quantities of blood-stained mucus, ranged from three to 10 per day. Most patients had little or no constitutional disturbances.

Although the dysentery may persist for weeks, it more commonly undergoes remissions and exacerbations and may eventually result in severe weight loss and prostration. In severe cases of amebic dysentery, symptoms may begin suddenly, diarrhea is profuse with 20 or more stools daily, and constitutional signs such as fever, dehydration, and electrolyte changes are usually seen.

Sigmoidoscopy reveals characteristic features in about 25% of patients. The earliest gross lesion is an ulcer the size of a pin head with hyperemic margins and slight edema of the surrounding mucosa. The typical amebic ulcer varies in diameter from a few millimeters to 2 cm, is shallow, is covered by a yellowish exudate, and has raised undermined edges. Although the ulcers are usually surrounded by a hyperemic margin, the intervening mucosa appears normal, except in severe cases in which mucosal edema and hyperemia may be generalized. The most common local complications of intestinal amebiasis are perforation and peritonitis, hemorrhage, strictures, and ameboma (a mass, most commonly found in the ileocecal region, consisting of inflamed, thickened intestinal wall surrounded by granulation tissue).

(2) Hepatic amebiasis. The diffuse enlargement of the liver which has been reported in association with acute intestinal dysentery does not have a direct amebic etiology. Abscesses, therefore, are now considered to be the only distinct clinical and pathological entity resulting from amebic infection of the liver. Sixty percent of patients with hepatic amebic abscess usually have no bowel symptoms, while the remainder may have nonspecific abdominal complaints. *E. histolytica* cysts or trophozoites are found in the stools in only 10% of patients. Of those who develop amebic liver abscess, about 50% may recollect a previous history of dysentery. Only in a small proportion of patients is amebic liver abscess found during acute intestinal amebiasis.

The onset of symptoms may be sudden or gradual. Pain in the right hypochondrium is the most striking symptom and is associated with fever ranging from 38 C to 39 C. Less commonly, cough, sweating, and loss of weight may be seen. The most characteristic finding on physical examination is tender hepatomegaly. Jaundice is exceedingly rare. There are also frequent changes at the base of the right lung, including impaired percussion note and diminished air entry due to elevation and immobility of the diaphragm. Laboratory examination usually shows a normal or slightly elevated white blood cell count, a normal level of serum bilirubin, and only a slight rise in level of liver enzymes. Liver scan should be performed and in most cases reveals the approximate size and location of the abscess. The majority of patients (87%) have single abscesses in the right lobe of the liver. The most common complication of liver abscess is rupture into the peritoneum or the thorax and through the skin. This situation has a grave prognosis.

Diagnosis

The process involved in the diagnosis of intestinal amebiasis is illustrated in figure 1. Amebiasis is first suspected on the basis of its presenting clinical features. Geographic history is particularly helpful since the infection is most prevalent in areas with poor hygienic conditions. Furthermore, amebic disease seems to occur more frequently in certain areas such as Mexico, South Africa, and India. A definitive diagnosis can be made by examination of stool specimens or bowel wall scrapings for *E. histolytica* cysts or trophozoites.

It is extremely important to realize, however, that the demonstration of *E. histolytica* trophozoites or cysts in fresh specimens of stools usually requires an experienced technician. It is necessary, therefore, to preserve a sample of the feces in polyvinyl alcohol. (PVA powder and PVA fixative solution may be purchased from Delkote, Inc., Pens Grove, N.J.) A freshly passed stool specimen should be mixed thoroughly with three times its volume of PVA fixative. The fixed specimen will retain the morphological characteristics of trophozoites and cysts and will en-

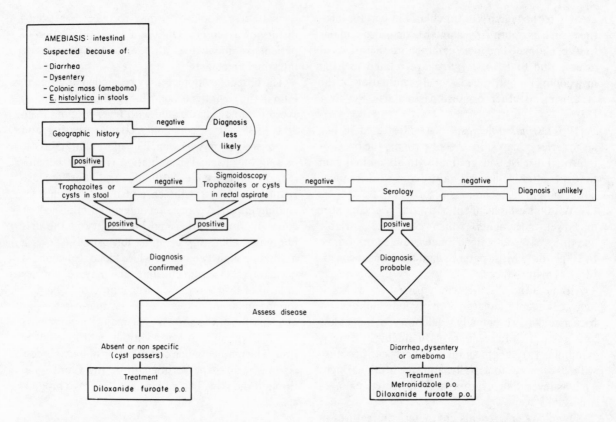

Figure 1. The progression to the diagnosis and treatment of intestinal amebiasis (*Entamoeba histolytica* infection); p.o. = perorally.

able shipment of the specimens for further identification procedures at state laboratories or the Center for Disease Control (CDC), Atlanta, Ga.

Microscopic examination of a wet mount of diarrheic or dysenteric stools within one-half hour after voiding, or of material obtained by scraping of the rectal mucosa during sigmoidoscopy, provides the best chance to demonstrate motile, red blood cell-containing trophozoites. Staining of stool smears by the Trichrome method [4] allows better definition of the morphological features of both trophozoites and cysts. In addition, a concentration technique such as the zinc sulfate method [4] may be helpful in the demonstration of amebic cysts. Examination of several stool samples is necessary if the infection is suspected, since excretion of cysts may be intermittent. The indirect HA test for amebiasis may be helpful as an adjunct in the diagnosis of acute amebic dysentery. Titers of ≥ 1:128 have been reported in 98% of cases [5].

In situations in which amebic liver abscess is suspected (figure 2), stool examination for the amebae is usually unrewarding. Under such circumstances, serological tests for antibodies to *E. histolytica* are particularly useful. The indirect HA test has been reported to be positive with a titer of ≥ 1:128 in virtually 100% of cases of amebic liver abscess [5]. The test is available at some state laboratories or at the CDC. Serum (1–2 ml) should be shipped at ambient temperature to state laboratories where they will be forwarded to the CDC if necessary. Positive serological results in the presence of signs and symptoms of liver abscess make the diagnosis highly probable. In most cases, however, it will be necessary to start treatment before receiving the results of the serological tests. Definitive diagnosis of amebic liver abscesses can be achieved only in cases in which aspiration is necessary as discussed below. The aspirate is odorless, brownish or pinkish in color, and free of bacteria on gram stain. Amebae may be found only in the last portion of aspirated material.

Management

As the factors responsible for the change of *E. histolytica* from the commensal mode of parasitism to

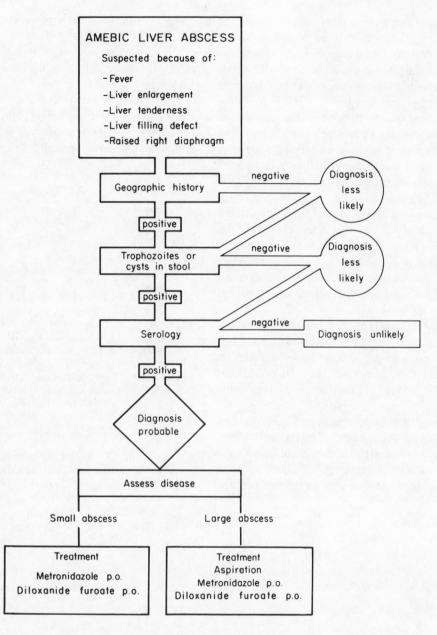

Figure 2.   The progression to the diagnosis and treatment of amebic liver abscess; p.o. = perorally.

the invasive forms are not clear, an attempt should be made to eliminate the organisms from the intestinal lumen of even asymptomatic persons who pass cysts [6]. Diloxanide furoate (obtained from the Parasitic Disease Drug Service of the Center for Disease Control, Atlanta, Georgia, tel. 404–633–3311) is the best lumenal amebicide presently available. The drug is highly effective against the trophozoites and cysts in the lumen of the gut but is ineffective against the tissue forms of the disease. The recommended dose

for adults is 500 mg orally three times daily for 10 days. The cure rate is >95%; however, it is recommended to re-examine stools 2–4 weeks following completion of therapy. Toxicity is rare, but mild abdominal discomfort may be encountered. The drug is not to be used for the treatment of pregnant women or children under two years of age.

Invasive amebiasis whether occurring in the intestines, the liver, or other organs necessitates the use of a tissue amebicide. Metronidazole (Flagyl,® Searle and Co., San Juan, Puerto Rico), which is now the drug of choice [7], is administered orally in a dose of 750 mg thrice daily for 10 days. Side effects include nausea, diarrhea, metallic taste in the mouth, dizziness, and sometimes discoloration of urine. Moderate leukopenia may occur occasionally, but the total white blood cell count returns to normal after completion of treatment. Alcohol should be avoided during the course of treatment because a confused state may occur. The drug is contraindicated in patients with blood dyscrasias or with active organic disease of the central nervous system. A course of diloxanide furoate, as described above, should follow treatment with metronidazole, which is relatively inefficient against the cyst stage of the parasite. Success of therapy should be evaluated by stool examination two weeks after completion of all amebicidal drug treatment, and the follow up of the regression of the liver abscess size by scans.

When oral therapy is not possible or metronidazole is contraindicated, the rapid and potent tissue amebicidal properties of dehydroemetine (obtained from the Parasitic Drug Service of the CDC; telephone number, 404-633-3311) may be life-saving. Dehydroemetine is administered sc or im (never iv) in a dose of 1 mg/kg of body weight and is limited to a maximal daily dose for adults of 60 mg for 10 days. The drug is cardiotoxic and should not be given to patients with heart or kidney disease. Patients given dehydroemetine should be kept on full bed rest and under constant medical supervision; the drug is discontinued at the first sign of cardiac toxicity (tachycardia, T-wave depression, or arrhythmias). A course of diloxanide furoate should also follow treatment with dehydroemetine.

Aspiration of a liver abscess is sometimes necessary for therapeutic purposes. The principal indications are lesions of >10 cm, evidence of imminent rupture, and poor clinical response after drug therapy for five days.

References

1. Osler, W. On the *Amoeba coli* in dysentery and in dysenteric liver abscess. Johns Hopkins Hosp. Bull. 1:53–54, 1890.
2. Juniper, K., Jr. Amebiasis in the United States. Bull. N.Y. Acad. Med. 47:448–461, 1971.
3. Wilmot, A. J. Clinical amoebiasis. F. A. Davis Co., Philadelphia, 1962. 166 p.
4. Melvin, D. M., Brooke, M. M. Laboratory procedures for the diagnosis of intestinal parasites. DHEW publication no. (CDC) 75-8282, U.S. Public Health Service, Center for Disease Control, Atlanta, Georgia, 1974, p. 79–131.
5. Kessel, J. F., Lewis, W. P., Pasquel, C. M., Turner, J. A. Indirect hemagglutination and complement fixation tests in amebiasis. Am. J. Trop. Med. Hyg. 14:540–550, 1965.
6. Mahmoud, A. A. F. Amebiasis. *In* H. F. Conn [ed.]. Current therapy. 1976. W. B. Saunders, Philadelphia, 1976, p. 2–3.
7. Cohen, H. G., Reynolds, T. B. Comparison of metronidazole and chloroquine for the treatment of amebic liver abscess. Gastroenterology 69:25–41, 1975.

Giardiasis

Giardiasis, a flagellate protozoan infection of the small bowel, has come into prominence during the last decade because of an increasing awareness that it may cause significant morbidity, the occurrence of localized outbreaks of epidemic proportions, and the importation of the infection by travelers. Infection with *Giardia lamblia* may be accompanied by persistent diarrhea and is sometimes associated with malabsorption. The infection is disseminated worldwide, with an average prevalence of 6.9%. In the United States giardiasis is both endemic and imported; the prevalence calculated from 24 published reports is 7.4% [1]. The epidemic nature of the infection has been noticed only recently. *G. lamblia* was the most commonly confirmed etiologic agent of outbreaks of waterborne diarrhea in the United States in 1974 [2]. Furthermore, during the last two years, sporadic cases or outbreaks have been reported in the Rocky Mountain states, Washington and New Hampshire [3, 4].

Imported giardiasis represents a considerable proportion of reported cases, particularly in travelers returning to the United States from Leningrad in the Soviet Union and from overland trips across the Middle East and the Indian subcontinent.

Life Cycle

G. lamblia resides in the upper part of the small intestine of man. The parasite exists in two forms, the trophozoite and the cyst. The trophozoite or active form is piriform in shape and usually measures $12–15 \times 5–15 \times 2–4$ μm. The body is bilaterally symmetrical; it is divided longitudinally by two slender median rods. Anteriorly, there are two oval nuclei, and the ventral aspect of the parasite includes a large concave sucking disk. There are also four pairs of flagella and a pair of characteristically curved median bodies that lie posterior to the sucking disk. The trophozoites are usually seen in duodenal aspirates and

in diarrheal but not in formed stools. The resistance of trophozoites to environmental conditions and the stimulus for encystation are unknown.

Giardial cysts are thick-walled and oval in shape, measuring $8–12 \times 7–10$ μm. Initially, they contain two nuclei, which divide into four nuclei in the mature cysts. The stools of infected individuals usually contain the cyst forms, which are the infective stage of the parasite. Cysts remain viable in water for longer than three months and have been shown to be infective after storage in tap water for 16 days.

Infection is spread either by direct fecal-oral contamination or by transmission of cysts in food or water. When ingested, the organisms excyst in the upper gastrointestinal tract and divide into two trophozoites, which mature in the duodenum and upper jejunum. Experimental infection was attempted by feeding cysts to volunteers; all of those who received 100–1,000,000 cysts became infected, 36.4% of those exposed to 10–25 cysts acquired the infection, and none exposed to just one cyst became infected.

Epidemiology

G. lamblia, the organism that naturally infects humans, has also been found in monkeys and pigs and has occasionally been transmitted to laboratory rats. Although different *Giardia* species are known to infect other animals, the question of host specificity is unsettled. If some *Giardia* species can be freely transmitted among different mammalian hosts, the possibility of an animal reservoir for human giardiasis or infection of humans with a species of *Giardia* that normally infects other animals must be considered.

The transmission of giardiasis has never been carefully examined. It is generally believed that the fecal-oral route is the mode of transmission, but no clear information is available on the usual vehicle. In the past, close proximity with infected individuals (as in institutions and boarding schools) was considered important. In recent outbreaks, however, waterborne transmission has been confirmed. The resistance of trophozoites to the external environment is unknown, but, by analogy with other protozoa, these relatively delicate forms are not considered to be a factor in the transmission of infection. Cysts, the infective stage of the organism, can live in fresh water for up to three months; the usual concentrations of chloramine, mercuric chloride, and formalin have no effect, but the cysts are killed by 2.5% phenol or lysol. With the exception of the house fly, a relatively inefficient transmitter of cysts, no other vehicles of transmission have been found.

Individuals vary in their response to *G. lamblia* infection. Whether this is due to differences in the virulence of the organism, to the strain or species of the parasite, or to host-related factors is a matter of considerable conjecture. Earlier studies have shown that childhood and malnutrition are associated with an increased prevalence of giardiasis. In addition, the association between symptomatic giardiasis and γ-globulin abnormalities has been suggested.

Disease Syndromes

G. lamblia infection may be asymptomatic, it may be associated with short-lived gastrointestinal symptomatology, or the disease may follow a prolonged intermittent course. The percentage of symptomatic patients varies from one study to another; it was as high as 55% in an epidemic and 80% in a group of patients examined for gastrointestinal complaints. The prevalence of symptomatology in surveys for endemic giardiasis appears to be far lower, suggesting some sort of acquired protection. Symptomatic patients may suffer from chronic diarrhea or malabsorption. Furthermore, a striking association between giardiasis and dysgammaglobulinemia has been observed recently.

(1) Chronic diarrhea. In contrast to bacterial diarrhea, the onset of giardial diarrhea is usually late, beginning one to three weeks after infection. The stools are loose, greasy, and sometimes watery. Although mucus is frequently seen in the stools, blood is rare. The diarrhea is often persistent, may be intermittent, and can be associated with marked weight loss. Patients may also complain of upper abdominal discomfort, bloating, and nausea.

(2) Malabsorption. With chronicity of the infection, steatorrhea and malabsorption may develop. Patients present with weight loss and bulky, greasy, foul-smelling stools that float in the toilet. Results of standard tests for malabsorption syndrome, such as fecal fat, D-xylose absorption, serum folate, and urinary excretion of vitamin B_{12}, are frequently abnormal. Nonspecific radiographic changes, such as thickening and distortion of mucosal folds, hypersecretion, and hypermotility, may be seen in the small intestine of these patients. Although most of the patients have structurally normal small bowel mucosa,

there may be evidence of acute and chronic inflammation, increased epithelial mitotic figures, abnormal configuration of the villi, or damage to epithelial cells. Careful examination of the mucosa has occasionally revealed invasive giardiae, but the significance of this phenomenon is not clear. The pathogenesis of diarrhea and steatorrhea is unknown. Possible factors include the creation of a mechanical barrier to absorption by massive growth of the organisms, competition between the parasite and the host for nutrients, and injury and invasion of the intestinal mucosa. Secretion of toxin by the organisms is another possible but unexplored mechanism.

(3) Giardiasis in dysgammaglobulinemia. Giardiasis has been implicated recently in the chronic diarrhea and malabsorption often noted in patients with dysgammaglobulinemia [5]. Most of these patients have low concentrations of serum IgA and IgM, with variable levels of IgG. The mucosal lesions are patchy and range from slight changes to severely disrupted villous architecture. Bacterial growth does not seem to be important in these patients, since broad-spectrum antibiotics are ineffective; improvement is achieved only through eradication of the parasite by specific treatment. It has recently been reported that congenitally athymic mice with markedly deficient cell-mediated immunological mechanisms are unable to clear *Giardia* infection similar to thymus-intact controls [6].

Diagnosis

The diagnosis and management of giardiasis is illustrated in the flow sheet in figure 1. Basic to this approach is the physician's awareness that giardiasis should be considered in the diagnosis of any patient with a diarrheal illness lasting one week or longer. Since giardiasis has a global distribution without a significant difference between the average prevalence in the United States and that in the rest of the world, a detailed geographic history of the patient will not be particularly helpful. An epidemiological history, however, linking the patient to a few localized areas of known infectivity (such as Leningrad and the Rocky Mountain states) or to diarrhea among travelers or campers may suggest the diagnosis.

Careful examination of stools is the next step in reaching the diagnosis. *G. lamblia* trophozoites or cysts in the stools can be detected by examination of direct smears. The sensitivity of stool examination can

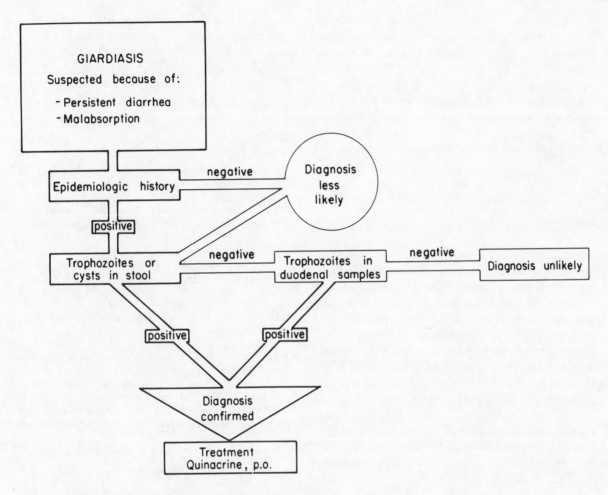

Figure 1.   The progression to a definitive diagnosis of giardiasis; p.o. = perorally.

be improved, however, by use of a concentration technique. The zinc sulfate concentration method is the simplest. (*1*) A suspension is prepared by mixing 1 g or 1 ml of stool with 10 ml of warm tap water. (*2*) The suspension is poured through a layer of damp gauze in a small funnel into a centrifuge tube, which is centrifuged for 2 min at 1,000 *g* (about 2,000 rpm). (*3*) The supernatant is decanted; water (3 ml) is added. The sediment is resuspended by shaking, and the tube is filled with water. This procedure is repeated until the supernatant becomes clear. (*4*) The supernatant is then poured off, and 3 ml of zinc sulfate solution (33 g/100 ml) is added, the sediment is resuspended, and more zinc sulfate solution is added, until the tube is filled to about 1.5 cm from the top. The tube is then centrifuged for 2 min at 2,000 *g* (about 3,000 rpm). (*5*) The surface film is transferred via a loop or pipette to a clean microscope slide, and two drops of iodine solution (1% potassium iodide

saturated with iodine) is added and mixed well. The slide is examined at × 100 magnification. Examination of several stool samples may be necessary, since excretion of the cysts is sometimes intermittent.

Negative stool findings necessitate sampling of duodenal contents either by intubation and aspiration or by the use of the recently described Enterotest (Hedeco, Palo Alto, Calif.) [7]. The device used consists of a gelatin capsule inside which is packed 140 cm of white nylon line. The capsule is swallowed by the patient and the free end of the line is secured to the face and left in position for 4 hr. In more than 95% of cases, the line extends to its full length and is carried into the duodenum by peristalsis. The line can be removed by gentle traction and its distal portion, which is saturated with bile-stained mucus, drawn through gloved fingers; a few drops of duodenal contents are expressed onto glass slides, which are examined immediately at × 100 magnification. In a recent study the capsule was found to be as successful in the diagnosis of giardiasis as duodenal intubation and had the added advantages of ease and convenience.

In cases in which all examinations yield negative results and intestinal biopsy is performed for general diagnostic purposes, the specimen should be briefly pressed onto a slide to obtain a mucosal impression smear, which can then be stained and examined for *G. lamblia*.

Management

The capacity of *G. lamblia* to multiply inside the human host and its potential pathogenicity make it imperative that all infected individuals, including those who are asymptomatic, be treated, and that treatment be curative, eradicating the parasitic flagellates. Quinacrine (mepacrine; Atabrine,® Winthrop Laboratories, New York, N.Y.) is the present drug of choice; a single oral course of 100 mg three times per day for 10 days provides a cure rate of more than 80% [8]. Toxicity of quinacrine in man is not marked and is mainly manifested as gastrointestinal (nausea, vomiting, colic) or mental symptoms (insomnia, confusion, psychosis). Failure of quinacrine therapy may necessitate either a second course or the use of metronidazole (Flagyl,® Searle, Chicago, Ill.), a drug that is highly effective only if used in larger doses than those usually recommended (i.e., 750 mg orally three times per day for 10 days).

References

1. Levine, N. D. *In* Protozoan parasites of domestic animals and of man. 2nd ed. Burgess Publishing, Minneapolis, 1973, p. 118–122.
2. Horwitz, M. A., Hughes, J. M., Craun, G. F. from the Center for Disease Control, Outbreaks of waterborne disease in the United States, 1974. J. Infect. Dis. 133:588–592, 1976.
3. Center for Disease Control. Morbidity and Mortality Weekly Rep. 23:78–79. 397–398. 1974.
4. Center for Disease Control. Morbidity and Mortality Weekly Report. 26:169–170, 1977.
5. Hoskins, L. C., Winawer, S. J., Broitman, S. A., Gottlieb, L. S., Zamcheck, N. Clinical giardiasis and intestinal malabsorption. Gastroenterology 53:265–279, 1967.
6. Stevens, D. P., Frank, D. M. and Mahmoud, A. A. F. Thymus dependency of host resistance to *Giardia muris* infection: studies in nude mice. J. Immunol. 120:680–682, 1978.
7. Beal, C. B., Viens, P., Grant, R. G. L., Hughes, J. M. A new technique for sampling duodenal contents. Demonstration of upper small bowel pathogens. Am. J. Trop. Med. Hyg. 19:349–352. 1970.
8. Petersen, H. Giardiasis (lambliasis). Scand. J. Gastroenterol. 14 (Suppl.):1–44, 1972.

Leishmaniases

The leishmaniases are zoonoses caused by intracellular protozoan parasites of the genus *Leishmania* which are transmitted to man by phlebotomine sandflies. When man is infected a spectrum of clinical conditions may occur, varying from localized or disseminated cutaneous and mucocutaneous lesions to generalized visceral leishmaniasis. The leishmaniases are endemic in many areas of the world, and it has recently been estimated that 12 million individuals have different forms of this protozoan infection.

Leishmania invade the reticuloendothelial cells, and the resulting disease is determined both by the parasite species and by the host response [1]. In central Asia, India, the Mediterranean littoral, and West Africa, cutaneous leishmaniasis or "Oriental sore" is caused by *Leishmania tropica*. In Central and South America, *Leishmania mexicana* and *Leishmania braziliensis* infections result in cutaneous ulcers that may spread to mucous membranes and cause severely mutilating facial lesions, e.g., "chiclero ulcer" and "espundia." Visceral leishmaniasis or "kala azar" results from infection with *Leishmania donovani* and is endemic in parts of China, the Indian subcontinent, the Mediterranean littoral, East Africa, and South America [2].

In the United States, three cases of autochthonous dermal leishmaniasis have been reported in Texas with serological evidence of infections due to *Leishmania* in dogs from the same area [3]. A total of several hundred cases of visceral leishmaniasis have been reported in the United States: in troops returning from World War II, in immigrants from endemic areas, and in individuals bitten by phlebotomine flies while traveling or residing in endemic areas; a few cases of visceral leishmaniasis have been found in dogs imported from Greece. Transmission of *L. donovani* infection to man, however, has not been reported in the United States.

Life Cycle

Organisms belonging to the genus *Leishmania* occur in two major forms, both of which multiply by binary fission [4], in their mammalian and insect hosts. In man and other mammals, the oval or rounded amastigotes (so called because they lack a flagellum) measure $4 \times 2 \ \mu$m and are usually found in the cells of the mononuclear phagocyte system but may also be seen in other peripheral blood leukocytes. When sandflies of the genus *Phlebotomus* obtain a blood meal from infected individuals or animals, they ingest the amastigotes. In the midgut of the insect, these organisms change to spindle-shaped promastigotes (so called because the flagellum passes directly out of the organism) which measure $17 \times 3 \ \mu$m. The promastigotes increase in number and, within four to five days, extend to the foregut of the insect. The promastigotes are transmitted to the mammalian host via the bite of the sandfly.

Epidemiology

Leishmaniasis is usually a zoonosis transmitted mainly by species of sandflies. These insects are abundant in the drier areas of the tropics and subtropics but may also be found in relatively humid areas. Only female sandflies take blood; they usually bite at night and shelter in dark corners by day.

In India and China, leishmaniasis is widespread throughout rural areas. In other regions where the disease is endemic, however, transmission is focal and may be related to environment as well as to relationships among animal reservoirs, vectors, and man. The dog is the principal animal reservoir for cutaneous and visceral leishmaniasis in many parts of the world, but gerbils and other wild rodents have also been found to play a role in transmission of the infection to man. Visceral leishmaniasis in India is the only form of the disease where there is no reported animal reservoir.

Although the organisms of the genus *Leishmania* that are infective for man are similar morphologically, they can be differentiated on the basis of the markedly different disease syndromes that are produced. Infection by a particular species of *Leishmania* is usually followed by long-lasting immunity to that species but not to others. All age groups and both sexes appear to be equally susceptible to infection with *Leishmania,* but in the Mediterranean basin the disease occurs largely in children. A fairly solid immunity follows infection with *L. tropica* in man. This has formed the basis of prophylactic inoculation which is being successfully practiced in Russia and the Middle East. It is noteworthy that immunization against cutaneous leishmaniasis probably represents the only known practical prophylaxis against a parasitic infection.

Disease Syndrome

(1) Cutaneous leishmaniasis of the Old World. "Oriental sore." The typical lesions, which may be single or multiple, commonly occur on the face, arms, and legs and appear two to eight weeks following sandfly bites. Lesions begin as small erythematous papules (2–5 mm in diameter), which enlarge slowly and may attain a size of 1–2 cm. Within a few months the nodules can develop into ulcers that remain as such for periods of up to two years, followed by slow healing and scar formation. Disseminated cutaneous leishmaniasis, apparently due to failure of the host's immune response, has been reported from Ethiopia.

(2) Cutaneous leishmaniasis of the New World, "chiclero ulcer" and "espundia." Many local names have been given to the cutaneous and mucocutaneous lesions of leishmaniasis in the New World, the most common being, respectively, "chiclero ulcer" and "espundia." The cutaneous lesions are similar to those seen in the Old World but are usually less nodular and more ulcerative. In "espundia" the lesions may spread to the mucocutaneous borders of the nose and mouth and erode into the nasal septum, resulting in gross facial deformity [5].

(3) Visceral leishmaniasis, "kala azar." The clinical syndrome produced by infection with *L. donovani* is due to invasion of the reticuloendothelial cells in the spleen, liver, bone marrow, lymph nodes, and skin. In the African and central Asian forms of the infection, a cutaneous nodule often develops at the site of the parasite inoculation within a few days and lasts for months. After an incubation period of two to six months, systemic manifestations usually develop insidiously. The earliest symptom is fever, which in >80% of cases develops into a characteristic pattern with twice-daily elevations in temperature. Other less common symptoms are dizziness, weakness, and weight loss. On physical examination the most characteristic sign of visceral leishmaniasis is enlargement of the spleen, which is firm, nontender, and may reach to the right iliac fossa. Lymphadenopathy, which may be generalized, is commonly seen in patients from Africa, the Mediterranean littoral, and China. Untreated infections become chronic and are complicated by anemia, bleeding tendencies, jaundice, and hypoalbuminemia; the mortality rate is 75%–90% and is due to intercurrent infections such as pneumonia and pulmonary tuberculosis. Laboratory examinations reveal anemia and leukopenia with agranulocytosis; thrombocytopenia is occasionally seen. The total serum concentration of protein is raised to >10 g/100 ml of serum almost entirely because of an increase in IgG.

Diagnosis

The progression to a diagnosis of visceral leishmaniasis is shown in figure 1. The infection should be suspected in individuals presenting with characteristic symptoms and signs who have migrated from or visited an area where leishmaniasis is endemic. A definitive diagnosis can be made by obtaining material for microscopic examination from the skin, bone marrow, or spleen.

When cutaneous or mucocutaneous leishmaniasis is suspected, examination of scrapings from slit skin smears taken from unulcerated parts of the lesions should be performed. The slit must be deep enough to reach the dermis but not to cause bleeding. In the case of visceral leishmaniasis, examination of bone marrow or spleen aspiration is the diagnostic step of choice. Several smears should be prepared, air-dried, and stained with Giemsa (Fisher Scientific Co., Fairtown, N.J.). The characteristic Leishman-Donovan bodies (amastigotes) can be seen within the macrophages, but these cells may rupture, and free organisms may be visualized. In circumstances in which the diagnosis is suspected but the smears obtained are negative, the aspirated material may be grown on diphasic blood agar medium [6] incubated at 22 C for three weeks. Alternatively, the aspirate may be inoculated ip into hamsters; amastigotes may be found in the spleens after two weeks.

Management

The only drug available in the United States for treatment of all forms of leishmaniasis, sodium antimony gluconate, can be obtained from the Center

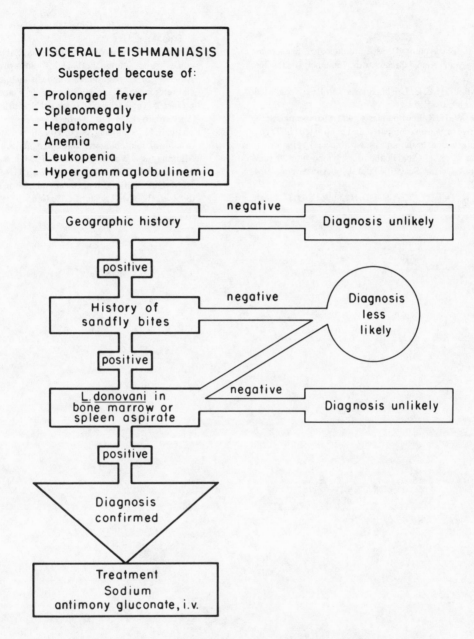

VISCERAL LEISHMANIASIS
Suspected because of:

- Prolonged fever
- Splenomegaly
- Hepatomegaly
- Anemia
- Leukopenia
- Hypergammaglobulinemia

Geographic history — negative → Diagnosis unlikely

positive

History of sandfly bites — negative → Diagnosis less likely

positive

L. donovani in bone marrow or spleen aspirate — negative → Diagnosis unlikely

positive

Diagnosis confirmed

Treatment
Sodium
antimony gluconate, i.v.

Figure 1. The progression to the diagnosis and management of visceral leishmaniasis.

for Disease Control, Atlanta, Ga. 30333. For adults a daily iv dose of 6 ml (100 mg of antimony/ml) is administered; the daily dose for children younger than 14 years is 4 ml and that for infants younger than two years is 2 ml. A course of six injections is given for visceral leishmaniasis acquired in India, 10 injections for cutaneous leishmaniasis of the Old World, and 30 injections for all other geographic forms of visceral leishmaniasis and for cutaneous leishmaniasis of the New World [7]. Side effects, mainly cardiac and hepatic, may occasionally be encountered during treatment with sodium antimony gluconate. Some forms of the mucocutaneous lesions of the New World may not respond to treatment with antimony compounds and require careful parenteral treatment with amphotericin B [7].

References

1. Turk, J. L., Bryceson, A. D. M. Immunological phenomena in leprosy and related diseases. Adv. Immunol. 13:209–266, 1971.
2. Manson-Bahr, P. E. C. Leishmaniasis. Int. Rev. Trop. Med. 4:123–139, 1971.
3. Lumsden, W. H. R. Leishmaniasis and trypanosomiasis: the causative organisms compared and contrasted. *In* Trypanosomiasis and leishmaniasis with special reference to Chagas' disease. Ciba Foundation Symposium 20 (new series). Associated Scientific Publishers, Amsterdam, 1974, p. 3–21.
4. Shaw, P. K., Quigg, L. T., Allain, D. S., Juranek, D. D., Healy, G. R. Autochthonous dermal leishmaniasis in Texas. Am. J. Trop. Med. Hyg. 25:788–796, 1976.
5. Convit, J. E., Pinardi, M. E. Cutaneous leishmaniasis: the clinical and immunopathological spectrum in South America. *In* Trypanosomiasis and leishmaniasis with special reference to Chagas' disease. Ciba Foundation Symposium 20 (new series). Associated Scientific Publishers, Amsterdam, 1974, p. 159–166.
6. Lennette, E. H., Spaulding, E. H., Truante, J. P. [ed.]. Manual of clinical microbiology. 2nd ed. American Society for Microbiology, Washington, D.C., 1974, p. 616.
7. Manson-Bahr, P. E. C. Leishmaniasis. *In* B. G. Maegraith and H. M. Gilles [ed.]. Management and treatment of tropical diseases. Blackwell Scientific, Oxford, 1971, p. 206–225.

Malaria

Malaria is a protozoal infection of man caused by four species of *Plasmodium: falciparum, vivax, ovale,* and *malariae.* These species are transmitted by female anopheline mosquitoes. Despite the well-publicized efforts to eradicate malaria, it still remains endemic in the humid, warm areas of the world, including most countries of Central and South America, Africa, and Asia. All four species of *Plasmodium* commonly cause fever and chills, anemia, and splenomegaly. *P. falciparum* differs importantly from the others, however, in that it is capable of causing high-density parasitemia which can progress rapidly to massive hemolysis and fatal cerebral and renal complications.

In the United States at the present time, most cases of malaria are found in travelers recently exposed to mosquitoes in endemic areas. In addition, transmission may occur by blood transfusion or by shared needles and syringes of drug addicts. The infection is rarely caused congenitally or by mosquito transmission from imported cases of malaria. The cardinal symptoms of acute malaria, chills and fever, are seen in so many common infections in the United States that American physicians rarely consider the diagnosis of malaria. Consequently, delays often occur and result in fatalities in patients with *P. falciparum* infections. This failure of physicians to consider the diagnosis appears to be largely responsible for the recent mortality rate of 8.5% for malaria in American civilian hospitals contrasted with a rate of only 0.7% in military hospitals [1]. Another important, but often neglected, responsibility of physicians in the United States is to advise travelers to endemic areas to have chemoprophylaxis for prevention of malaria.

Life Cycle

Parasites that cause malaria undergo a series of complex morphological changes associated with marked multiplication of the organisms during their passage in man and in insect vectors. Man is infected by the bite of female anopheline mosquitoes, which inject saliva containing the infective sporozoite forms. After circulating for <30 min in the blood, the sporozoites enter the liver parenchymal cells where they multiply. Seven to 10 days later, multiple small forms break out of the hepatocytes into the bloodstream and enter red blood cells. Dormancy of the infection in the liver parenchymal cells explains relapses in malaria caused by *P. vivax* and *P. ovale.* Although *P. malariae* and *P. falciparum* infections have been shown to lack the mechanism of dormancy, persistence of low-level parasitemia has been shown in *P. malariae* infections.

In the red blood cells, the organisms grow from the so-called ring forms (as seen in stained blood smears) through different morphological stages and then divide into multiple infective merozoites. After breaking out of the erythrocytes, the merozoites enter new red blood cells. The length of this cycle is two days for *P. vivax, P. ovale,* and *P. falciparum* and three days for *P. malariae* and is manifested clinically by the characteristic periodicity of the febrile attacks. After a few of these cycles, some merozoites change into sexual forms (gametocytes), which on ingestion by mosquitoes complete the life cycle.

In the stomach of the mosquito, the male microgametocytes emit a series of six to eight flagellae. These break free and, on encountering the female macrogametes penetrate into them. The fertilized zygotes enter the stomach wall where they multiply into massive numbers of infective sporozoites. The sporozoites then break out into the body cavity and migrate to the salivary glands. The development of the parasite in the mosquito is completed in 10–21 days, depending on the species of *Plasmodium* and the ambient temperature.

In malaria induced by transfusion or by needles and syringes shared by drug addicts, red blood cells containing the parasites enter the blood directly, initiating the erythrocytic cycle. Since there is no hepatic stage, relapses do not occur.

Epidemiology

Naturally transmitted malaria has been eradicated in the United States, most of Europe, Japan, and Australia. However, malaria remains endemic in the countries designated in table 1 in those areas where there are anopheline vectors and a human reservoir

Table 1. Countries reporting transmission of malaria to the World Health Organization in 1973.

General area	Specific area
Africa	All countries except Lesotho and the islands of Mauritius and Réunion.
Central America and Caribbean islands	All countries. Haiti and Dominican Republic reported malaria but other Caribbean islands are malaria-free.
South America	All countries except Chile and Uruguay.
Europe, including Turkey and the Soviet Union	Limited foci only in Greece, Turkey, and the Soviet Union.
Asia, west of the Indian subcontinent	All countries except Cyprus, Israel, and Lebanon.
Indian subcontinent	All countries.
Eastern Asia and Oceania	All countries except Australia, Hong Kong, Japan, Macao, New Zealand, and certain Pacific islands.

NOTE. For further details concerning *Plasmodium* species that cause malaria and areas within countries that are malaria-free, see [2, 3].

of infection. Within these countries large cities are often malaria-free, and, at high altitudes and at certain times of year, malaria is not transmitted [2, 3]. All four species of *Plasmodium* exist together in most endemic regions, but *P. vivax* and *P. falciparum* cause the great majority of cases of malaria reported in the world; *P. malariae* is less common, and *P. ovale* is exceedingly rare.

Malaria caused by chloroquine-resistant *P. falciparum* was discovered in Colombia in 1961. Since that time, the number of countries reporting chloroquine resistance has expanded to include those in table 2 [2]. This problem has not appeared in Africa and does not occur in species other than *P. falciparum*.

All ages, sexes, and races appear to be equally susceptible to malaria, except for blacks with sickle cell trait, who have partial protection against falciparum malaria, and for many blacks lacking certain Duffy blood group determinants, who are protected against *P. vivax* infections. The risk of developing malaria is greatest for persons heavily exposed to mosquitoes, particularly if they have not had prophylaxis for malaria.

Now that the Vietnam conflict has ended, there is again a preponderance of civilian over military cases

of malaria in the United States (302:21 in 1974). The civilians were most commonly tourists, businessmen, college teachers and students, and missionaries who had arrived from countries endemic for malaria. The identified infecting species were *P. vivax* (51%), *P. falciparum* (29%), *P. malariae* (8%), and *P. ovale* (3%). The time after arrival in the United States that patients became ill was shortest for *P. falciparum*. In 1974, 82% of all patients infected with *P. falciparum* were diagnosed within one month after arrival, whereas only 35% of the *P. vivax* infections occurred in the first month. Only 1% of patients infected with *P. falciparum* developed illness after six months from the time of arrival, whereas 17%–28% of patients infected with the other three species of *Plasmodium* became ill after six months or more [4]. Asymptomatic parasitemia caused by *P. malariae* may be detected several years after arrival in the United States and can be a source of transfusion-induced infections.

Within the United States in 1974, there were three instances of transfusion-induced malaria and one patient with congenitally transmitted infection, all caused by *P. malariae*. There were three cases of mosquito-transmitted malaria, which were caused by *P. vivax*. Six fatalities occurred during that year, and all were due to *P. falciparum* [4].

Disease Syndromes

The common presenting symptoms of malaria are chills and fever. The onset is usually sudden, with a violently shaking chill followed by a marked rise in temperature; profuse sweating then occurs. During the first few days, fever may either occur irregularly or be continuous. Subsequently, the febrile paroxysms may become periodic with intervals between the episodes of 48 hr in *P. vivax, P. falciparum,* and *P. ovale* infections and 72 hr in *P. malariae* infections. In *P. falciparum* malaria, however, the cycles of fever tend to be unpredictable, with either more than one fever spike per day or a continuous high fever. At times, the onset of the infection is insidious, with low-grade fever. Rarely, malaria may be seen without fever and with protean manifestations such as diarrhea, abdominal pain, dyspnea, headache, or myalgia. The spleen is palpable in most patients. Anemia may be mild or absent in an early attack, but some patients with *P. falciparum* malaria have rapid hemolysis with severe anemia and jaundice. The white blood cell counts are usually normal or low.

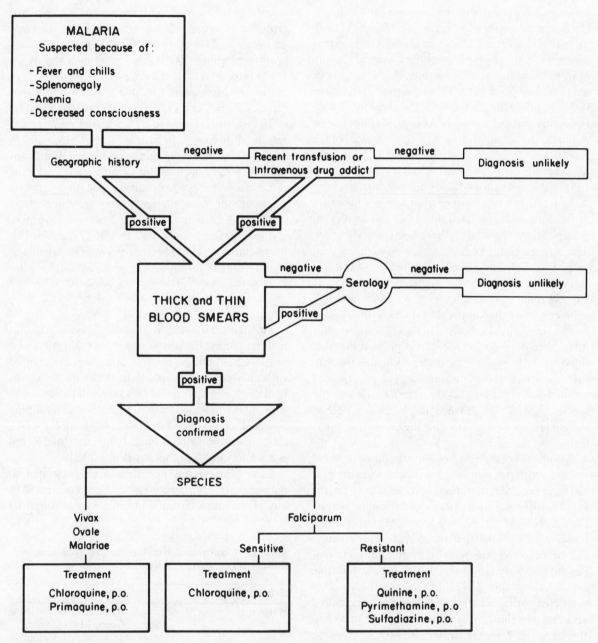

Figure 1.   The progression to the diagnosis and treatment of malaria; p.o. = perorally. Primaquine is only necessary in the treatment of infections due to *Plasmodium vivax* and *Plasmodium ovale*.

Malaria caused by *P. vivax* and *P. ovale* may relapse with recurrent episodes of fever for a period of months or years, whereas *P. falciparum* infections never relapse. However, falciparum malaria can rapidly advance to a high-density parasitemia with 5%->50% of red blood cells parasitized; this condition is associated with hemolysis and severe anemia. Acute renal failure may result from massive hemoglobinuria. A more ominous complication is cerebral malaria, which is associated with coma and a high mortality rate. *P. malariae* infections, in which there may be prolonged asymptomatic parasitemia, have been associated with development of the nephrotic syndrome.

Diagnosis

After malaria is suspected because of fever in a person

with a positive geographic history, in a recipient of a blood transfusion, or in a drug addict (iv use) (figure 1), both thin and thick blood smears must be prepared promptly. A thin smear is prepared by placing a drop of fresh blood on the end of a slide. With the edge of another slide placed at a 30° angle to the first slide, the front of the drop is touched, and the slanted slide is quickly pushed forward. After drying for a few minutes, the smear is dipped in methyl alcohol for fixation. As the density of parasites may be too low for detection on a thin smear (often less than one per 1,000 red blood cells), a thick smear is also necessary. A drop of fresh blood either from a finger puncture or from an anticoagulated tube is placed on a clean glass slide and spread with the corner of another slide over an area about 1 cm in diameter and dried at 37 C for 1 hr. Both slides are then stained with Giemsa stain (Fisher Scientific Co., Fairlawn, N.J.) [5]. If Giemsa is not available, however, a routine Wright's stain can be applied to the thin smear without prior fixation in methyl alcohol and to the thick smear after it has been dehemoglobinized by dipping it into distilled water to remove the color. Although the thin smear is more easily interpreted by inexperienced persons and is also useful for determination of the species, the thick smear when read by an experienced technician is more sensitive for the diagnosis of malaria.

A diagnosis of malaria frequently requires repeated smears at different times of the day because the parasitemia may be intermittent or its level may fluctuate. Multiple negative smears rule strongly against the diagnosis of malaria in a febrile patient. Rarely, however, cases of malaria with subpatent parasitemia can be detected serologically by the indirect fluorescent antibody (IFA) test, which is both sensitive and relatively specific [6]. In the case of a strongly suspected patient with negative blood smears, paired sera and unstained blood smears should be mailed to the Parasitic Diseases Branch, Center for Disease Control (CDC), Atlanta, Georgia 30333. Further advice can be obtained from the CDC by telephoning 404-633-3311. Titers of ≥1:16 indicate an active or recent (within six months) malaria infection [6] and should prompt the physician to repeat blood smear examinations.

Treatment

The choice of treatment for malaria depends on the

infecting species, mode of transmission, and place of probable infection. There are only three different regimens, and for every patient with malaria the appropriate regimen can be chosen as shown in figure 1. For infections caused by *P. vivax, P. ovale,* and *P. malariae* chloroquine phosphate (Winthrop Laboratories, New York, N.Y.) is given initially in a dose of 1 g perorally, followed by 0.5 g after 6 hr and 0.5 g daily for two days. In patients with *P. vivax* and *P. ovale* infections, primaquine phosphate (Winthrop) in a dose of 26.3 mg daily for 14 days is given after the chloroquine therapy to eradicate the latent parasitic stages in the liver. Patients who are infected by transfusion or shared needles, however, have only erythrocytic forms and do not require primaquine [7]. Primaquine can cause severe hemolysis in patients of Mediterranean origin with glucose-6-phosphate dehydrogenase (G6PD) deficiency, but causes only mild self-limited hemolysis in blacks with G6PD deficiency.

Falciparum malaria is a medical emergency that requires prompt therapy to prevent complications and death. Chloroquine-sensitive infections are treated with chloroquine phosphate in the same dosage as nonfalciparum infections. In severely ill patients who cannot take oral medication, parenteral chloroquine hydrochloride, which is available only from the CDC, should be administered im or iv in a dose of 250 mg every 6 hr until oral therapy is possible [8].

Chloroquine-resistance should be presumed in patients with *P. falciparum* infections contracted in any of the areas outlined in table 2 or acquired by

Table 2. Countries with malaria caused by chloroquine-resistant *Plasmodium falciparum.*

General area	Specific area
Western Hemisphere	Brazil (only Amazonas, Espirito Santo, Goias, Mato Grosso, Para, and Roraima), Colombia (not Bogota), Panama, Surinam, and Venezuela (only the southern areas, Bolivar, and Barinas).
Asia	Burma, Cambodia, India (only Assam and Meghalaya), Indonesia (only Kalimantan and western Irian), Laos, Malaysia, Nepal, Philippines (only the area of Manila and Palawan), Singapore, Thailand, and Vietnam.

blood transfusions or needles. The treatment of choice is 650 mg of quinine sulfate (Eli Lilly and Company, Indianapolis, Ind.) perorally three times daily for 14 days combined with 25 mg of pyrimethamine (Burroughs-Wellcome, Research Triangle Park, N.C.) perorally twice daily for three days and 500 mg of sulfadiazine (Eli Lilly) perorally four times daily for five days. In severely ill patients quinine hydrochloride can be given iv in a dose of 600 mg in 300 ml of saline over 30 min every 8 hr until oral therapy is possible. Pyrimethamine must be omitted in pregnant patients.

Patients presenting with complications of *P. falciparum* infections, such as acute renal failure, cerebral symptoms, or pulmonary edema, will need appropriate supportive therapy in addition to antimalarial therapy [9]. All patients with *P. falciparum* infections should have blood smears repeated daily to ensure that therapy has eliminated the parasites, because a resistant infection mistakenly treated with chloroquine can progress to a parasitemia of higher density or can recrudesce after initial improvement. Gametocytes may appear during treatment, but their presence does not indicate failure of therapy. Reappearance of fever within a month after treatment of malaria in the United States may mean a recrudescence of malaria. Accordingly, patients must be instructed to return for reexamination if fever should reappear.

Prevention

Most cases of malaria imported into the United States could be prevented if travelers going to malarious countries were advised to have chemoprophylaxis. A traveler intending to visit any of the countries listed in table 1 should take 500 mg of chloroquine phosphate weekly beginning one week before departure and continuing for six weeks after return. Since most cases of malaria in the United States are caused by *P. vivax* and since the incidence of these cases has recently increased [4], a traveler after returning from a malarious area should add to his regimen 26.3 mg of primaquine phosphate daily for 14 days.

A traveler going to countries reporting chloroquine-resistant falciparum malaria (table 2) must understand that chloroquine will provide only partial protection. Complete protection can be offered by the new drug pyrimethamine-sulfadoxine (Fansidar,® Roche Products Ltd., England), which is not available in the United States but can be obtained abroad. One tablet a week should be taken during exposure to malaria.

Protective measures against mosquito bites should be recommended to travelers. These measures include sleeping under mosquito netting or in screened houses, wearing long sleeves at night, spraying houses with insecticides, and applying mosquito repellents such as N,N,-diethyltoluamide (OFF,® S.C. Johnson and Son, Racine, Wis.) to exposed parts of the body [3].

References

1. Heineman, H. S. The clinical syndrome of malaria in the United States. A current review of diagnosis and treatment for American physicians. Arch. Intern. Med. 129:607–616, 1972.
2. Six-monthly information on the world malaria situation. Wkly. Epidem. Rec. 50:53–72, 1975.
3. Information on malaria risk for international travelers. Wkly. Epidem. Rec. 48:25–48, 1973.
4. Shaw, P. K., Brodsky, R. E., Shultz, M. G. Malaria surveillance in the United States, 1974. J. Infect. Dis. 133:95–101, 1976.
5. Shute, P. G. The staining of malaria parasites. Trans. R. Soc. Trop. Med. Hyg. 60:412–416, 1966.
6. Kagan, I. G., Matthews, H., Sulzer, A. J. The serology of malaria: recent applications. Bull. N.Y. Acad. Med. 45:1027–1042, 1969.
7. Miller, L. H. Transfusion malaria. *In* T. J. Greenwalt and G. A. Jamieson [ed.]. Transmissible disease and blood transfusion. Grune and Stratton, New York, 1975, p. 241–266.
8. Drugs for parasitic infections. *In* Handbook of antimicrobial therapy. The Medical Letter, New Rochelle, 1974, p. 60.
9. Miller, L. H. Malaria. *In* H. F. Conn [ed.]. Current therapy 1976. W. B. Saunders, Philadelphia, 1976, p. 36–38.

Toxoplasmosis

Infection with the intracellular protozoan parasite *Toxoplasma gondii* is widespread throughout the world. Toxoplasmosis acquired by adults is usually asymptomatic, although its most common clinical manifestation is an infectious mononucleosis-like syndrome. *T. gondii* infection may also be transmitted via the placenta, causing abortions, still births, or congenital abnormalities. Serologically, the prevalence of antibodies to *T. gondii* varies widely in different parts of the world, ranging between 1% and 70% with an estimated mean of 30% [1].

In various parts of the United States, serological surveys have shown the prevalence of *T. gondii* in adults to vary from 20% to 70% [1, 2]. Congenital toxoplasmosis has been estimated to occur at a rate of 0.25–5.0 cases per 1,000 live births. In adults, there is little accurate data on the incidence of disease due to *T. gondii* although it appears to be low. Recently, considerable morbidity and mortality due to toxoplasmosis have been observed in immunosuppressed individuals.

Life Cycle

T. gondii is an obligate intracellular protozoan which is ubiquitous in nature, infecting virtually all mammalian species. In the past, acquired infection appeared to occur solely by ingestion of raw or undercooked meat containing cysts of the parasite. The complete life cycle of *T. gondii,* which has only recently been discovered, appears to be confined to members of the cat family [3]. In these animals *T. gondii* is a coccidian-like parasite which multiplies within the epithelial lining of the jejunum, ileum, and colon. The feces of infected cats contain the oocyst forms (10 × 12 μm in size with a resistant wall), which become infective within four days. Ingestion of the infective oocysts by cats is followed by invasion of the intestinal epithelium and intracellular multiplication of the organisms within 12 hr.

Individuals infected by the oocysts from cat feces or cysts in meat may show a parasitemia in the acute stages of the infection. The parasitic forms that can be recovered from blood or tissues during this stage, and which are called trophozoites, are crescent-shaped and measure 3 × 7 μm. Later in the course of infection, *T. gondii* cysts containing numerous organisms appear in the tissues, particularly the brain and skeletal and heart muscles, where they remain for the life span of the host. Man can also be infected by transplacental transmission of the organisms when the mother acquires the infection during pregnancy.

Epidemiology

Toxoplasmosis is a zoonosis which has been found in numerous warm-blooded animals and birds. In many cases it appears to be transmitted by the consumption of raw or undercooked meat containing cysts, although oocysts in cat feces may also transmit toxoplasmosis to man and animals. Toxoplasma oocysts have been found to survive in soil for periods up to 18 months and appeared to persist longer in moist than in dry areas [4]. Insects such as flies and cockroaches may transport the oocysts to human food. Since the discovery of the resistant oocyst of *T. gondii* in feline feces, the extent of the role of cats in the epidemiology of toxoplasmosis has been recently investigated. Some studies have found that contact with pet cats is associated with a greater prevalence of antibodies to *T. gondii*, whereas other studies have not confirmed this association. Infection once established in the human host is lifelong, although only a small proportion of those infected develop overt disease.

Clinical Syndromes

The widespread prevalence of antibodies to *T. gondii* in human sera and the low incidence of recognizable disease suggest that infection is asymptomatic in the great majority of individuals [2]. In adults, several clinical syndromes resulting from *T. gondii* infection have been described.

(1) Acute toxoplasmosis. The most common presentation is localized lymphadenopathy, which may also be generalized. The enlarged lymph nodes usually are discrete and not tender, and in many cases

they are discovered accidentally by the patient. In a report of a large series of clinically overt toxoplasmosis, the most commonly involved lymph node group was the cervical followed by the suboccipital (10%) [5]. Enlargement of the lymph nodes was accompanied by fever in 40% of cases, hepatomegaly and splenomegaly in 33%, and sore throat in 20%. The major presenting symptoms were fever (40%), fatigue (40%), and maculopapular skin rash (10%). The syndrome of acute toxoplasmosis often resembles infectious mononucleosis, with absolute peripheral blood lymphocytosis and an occasional atypical lymphocyte. Rarely, *T. gondii* infections may end fatally due to encephalitis and/or pneumonia.

The question of acquired toxoplasmosis during pregnancy is of great medical significance [6]. The risk of placental transmission to the fetus apparently is related to the time during gestation when maternal infection occurs. Early in gestation, transmission to the fetus appears to be less frequent, but when it occurs the disease tends to be severe. Although transmission is more frequent late in gestation, the newborn usually develops inapparent infection or subclinical disease, and only months later severe untoward sequelae may appear, such as mental retardation, epilepsy, and ocular lesions.

(2) Ocular toxoplasmosis. Involvement of the eye may occur in both congenital and, less commonly, acquired toxoplasmosis. The characteristic pathology in these individuals is a focal necrotizing retinochoroiditis which may cause haziness of vision, pain, and photophobia. The lesions usually appear as small clusters of yellowish white cotton-like patches in the fundus. Less commonly, periuveitis, papillitis, or optic atrophy have been observed.

(3) Toxoplasmosis in the immunosuppressed host. Toxoplasmosis has been recognized as one of the important opportunistic infections in immunosuppressed patients, particularly those with lymphoma or leukemia [7, 8]. The infection in these individuals may be acquired with generalized symptoms or represents reactivation of a latent infection. In a series of 81 cases of disseminated toxoplasmosis in immunosuppressed individuals, >50% presented with signs and symptoms of generalized central nervous system involvement. Disturbances of consciousness, seizures, motor impairment, and abnormal reflexes were common. Localized neurological findings suggestive of space-occupying lesions were encountered less frequently. Signs of pulmonary or cardiac involvement may also be seen.

(4) Congenital toxoplasmosis. This form of toxoplasmosis is usually the result of asymptomatic acute infection in the mother. Spontaneous abortion, prematurity, and a host of clinical presentations have been associated with maternal transmission of *T. gondii* to the fetus. Detailed clinical descriptions are available [6, 9].

Diagnosis

The process involved in the diagnosis and management of acquired toxoplasmosis is illustrated in figure 1. From individuals presenting symptoms or signs suggestive of toxoplasmosis, an epidemiological history should be obtained stressing contact with cats and soil or consumption of undercooked meat. Although a positive history may suggest the possibility of toxoplasmosis, its absence does not rule out *T. gondii* infection. A probable diagnosis of toxoplasmosis depends on either serological evidence or characteristic histology of lymph nodes. The two most valuable serological tests involve the measurement of conventional and IgM fluorescent antibodies [1]; both tests are available from the Center for Disease Control. Serum samples (1–2 ml) should be sent at ambient temperature to state laboratories for forwarding to the Center for Disease Control. Titers of >1:1,000 in the conventional indirect fluorescent antibody assay suggest the possibility of acute infection. Since IgM antibodies appear earlier and disappear sooner than IgG antibodies, their presence suggests acute infection; a titer of ≥1:10 is considered positive.

The second most helpful diagnostic procedure is lymph node biopsy, since certain histological features of *Toxoplasma* infection are reportedly pathognomonic [10]. Reactive follicular hyperplasia is seen associated with irregular clusters of epithelioid histiocytes in the cortical and paracortial areas; these clusters characteristically encroach upon and blur the margins of the germinal centers. Epithelioid cells are frequently observed in the germinal centers. It should be realized that a definitive diagnosis is difficult in toxoplasmosis, as demonstration of the trophozoites in biopsy material or isolation of the organisms after animal inoculation is rarely successful.

Management

The decision to treat patients with active toxoplasmosis depends on the degree of activity of the infec-

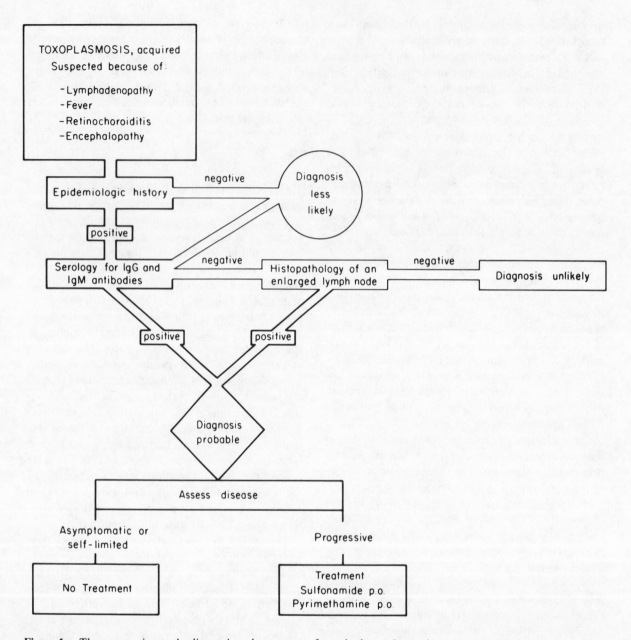

Figure 1. The progression to the diagnosis and treatment of acquired toxoplasmosis; p.o. = perorally.

tion and extent of the disease. Therapy is necessary in acute toxoplasmosis with systemic manifestations, in the infected immunosuppressed host, in cases with active ocular lesions, and in infected newborns whether or not they are symptomatic [6]. Treatment of mild cases, however, is unnecessary. A combination of pyrimethamine and sulfadiazine is used: pyrimethamine is given orally in a loading dose of 100 mg on day 1 followed by 25 mg daily for six weeks. The first oral dose of sulphadiazine is 4 g, followed by 1

g four times daily for six weeks. Since pyrimethamine is an inhibitor of the enzyme dihydrofolate reductase and bone marrow suppression may occur, folinic acid should be added in a daily dose of 6 mg, and regular blood counts should be performed. Fulminant cases of ocular toxoplasmosis may necessitate the addition of corticosteroids to reduce the inflammatory response. Prevention of toxoplasmosis depends on breaking the transmission chain to man [11]. Children and pregnant women constitute two high-risk groups who should avoid eating undercooked or raw meat and exercise particular care after handling raw meat, soil, or cats.

References

1. Anderson, S. E., Jr., Remington, J. S. Current concepts in diagnosis: the diagnosis of toxoplasmosis. South. Med. J. 68:1433–1443, 1975.
2. Warren, K. S., Dingle, J. H. A study of illness in a group of Cleveland families. XXII. Antibodies to *Toxoplasma gondii* in 40 families observed for ten years. N. Engl. J. Med. 274:993–997, 1966.
3. Jacobs, L. *Toxoplasma gondii:* parasitology and transmission. Bull. N.Y. Acad. Med. 50:192–210, 1974.
4. Frenkel, J. K., Ruiz, A., Chinchilla, M. Soil survival of *Toxoplasma* oocysts in Kansas and Costa Rica. Am. J. Trop. Med. Hyg. 24:439–443, 1975.
5. Kean, B. H. Clinical toxoplasmosis–50 years. Trans. R. Soc. Trop. Med. Hyg. 66:549–567, 1972.
6. Remington, J. S., Desmont, S. G. Toxoplasmosis. *In* J. S. Remington and J. O. Klein [ed.]. Infectious diseases of the fetus and newborn infant. W. B. Saunders, Philadelphia, 1976, p. 191–332.
7. Frenkel, J. K., Nelson, B. M., Arias-Stella, J. Immuno-suppression and toxoplasmic encephalitis: clinical and experimental aspects. Hum. Pathol. 6:97–111, 1975.
8. Ruskin, J., Remington, J. S. Toxoplasmosis in the compromised host. Ann. Intern. Med. 84:193–199, 1976.
9. Alford, C. A., Stagno, S., Reynolds, D. W. Congenital toxoplasmosis: clinical, laboratory, and therapeutic considerations, with special reference to subclinical disease. Bull. N.Y. Acad. Med. 50:160–181, 1974.
10. Dorfman, R. F., Remington, J. S. Value of lymph node biopsy in the diagnosis of acute acquired toxoplasmosis. N. Engl. J. Med. 289:878–881, 1973.
11. Frenkel, J. K. Breaking the transmission chain of *Toxoplasma*: a program for the prevention of human toxoplasmosis. Bull. N.Y. Acad. Science 50:228–235, 1974.

African Trypanosomiases

The human trypanosomiases of Africa are infections caused by two subspecies of the hemoflagellate *Trypanosoma brucei: T. brucei rhodesiense* and *T. brucei gambiense*; these subspecies are transmitted to man through the bite of tsetse flies of the genus *Glossina*. Although the two subspecies are morphologically indistinguishable, they differ epidemiologically and in their disease spectrum. Infection with *T. brucei rhodesiense* often results in a subacute fatal disease, whereas infection with *T. brucei gambiense* usually runs a more chronic course, manifested clinically by the typical sleeping sickness syndrome. The human trypanosomiases are transmitted in the region of Africa between 15° N and 15° S latitude, where the environmental conditions correspond to those favorable for glossina flies [1]. The rhodesian form of the infection occurs largely in the eastern third of Central Africa, whereas the gambian infection is found mainly in the western half of this region. Data on the prevalence of the infections during the last two decades are grossly incomplete at present because of a decrease in surveillance and control activities.

The possibility of acquiring trypanosomiasis while traveling in Africa has recently been emphasized. During the period 1967–1974, nine cases of African trypanosomiasis were diagnosed and treated in Americans, six in the United States and three abroad [2]. With the increase in international travel, 20,000 Americans are now estimated to visit endemic areas yearly. In addition, about 10,000 aliens enter the United States each year from countries in Africa where the infection is endemic. The African trypanosomiases range from acute to chronic diseases and, if untreated, almost invariably terminate in death. Another problem with these infections is that the drugs for treating them are highly toxic and must be used with great caution.

Life Cycle

T. brucei rhodesiense and *T. brucei gambiense* undergo several morphological changes during their life cycle through the human or vertebrate host and the insect vector [3]. Human infection is acquired through the bite of tsetse flies, in which the infective metacyclic forms of the organisms (15 μm long and without a free flagellum) enter the skin in the saliva of the insect. Within two to three days, these forms change into long thin forms, and, after local multiplication in the skin, they disseminate to the peripheral blood and lymph one to three weeks after inoculation. The central nervous system may be invaded early in the course of the rhodesian infection (weeks) but is delayed (months) in the gambian form. The forms in the bloodstream, known as trypomastigotes, are typically polymorphic, varying from long and slender (mean length, 28 μm) through intermediate to stumpy forms (mean length, 20 μm). The slender forms, which possess a free flagellum and a well-developed undulating membrane, are usually predominant; they are the only form in the blood that shows an appreciable rate of binary division.

The insect vectors are species of tsetse flies of the genus *Glossina* that vary with the subspecies of trypanosome and the endemic area. Both male and female flies are hematophagous and potentially infectible, but only a small portion of them become infected on ingestion of a blood meal from an infected individual. Initially, the organisms localize in the posterior part of the midgut, where they multiply into slightly modified trypomastigotes. After 10–12 days they begin to migrate anteriorly to the proventriculus and then to the salivary glands of the flies where they multiply further and change into infective metacyclic forms. The life cycle in the tsetse flies is completed in 15–35 days. Contrary to the above so-called "cyclic transmission" of trypanosomiases by the tsetse flies, mechanical transmission directly by the mouth parts of the insect may take place, but this phenomenon has been observed only during epidemics. In addition, congenital transmission of trypanosomes from mothers to their infants has been reported.

Epidemiology

A major factor in the epidemiology of African trypanosomiasis is the relative inefficiency of the insect vector. *Glossina* species captured in endemic areas show a low prevalence of infection (≤4.8%), and in the laboratory ≤10% of the flies sustain the development of the infective forms after being fed trypanosomes. Moreover, tsetse flies are susceptible to the infection only during the first four days after their emergence from the pupal stage.

Although *T. brucei rhodesiense* and *T. brucei gambiense* are morphologically indistinguishable, they differ markedly in their epidemiology and their virulence to the mammalian host. The species of tsetse flies that transmit *T. brucei rhodesiense* live in vast, relatively sparsely inhabited areas of the East African plains. The rhodesian organisms produce an acute, often fatal disease in humans, thereby reducing the chance of transmission to the insect vector. A nonhuman reservoir for the maintenance of the trypanosome life cycle is thus necessary, and *T. brucei rhodesiense* has been isolated from both the bushbuck and the hartebeest.

The *Glossina* species transmitting the gambian form of the infection inhabit the forested banks of rivers and similar humid areas. Important foci of transmission are found where people habitually cross rivers or enter them to wash or to collect water. *T. brucei gambiense* produces a chronic disease, and this fact, plus the greater frequency of biting by the species of tsetse fly that transmits this form of the infection than that of the rhodesian organism, may explain the continuation of its life cycle in the absence of demonstrable animal reservoirs.

Disease Syndromes

(1) Acute African trypanosomiasis. In both types of trypanosomiasis, but more often in the rhodesian form, an entry lesion, the trypanosomal nodule or "chancre," may be noticed two or three days after the tsetse bite. In four to 10 days, the lesion becomes a small, hard, painful, red nodule surrounded by a relatively larger zone of erythema and swelling; the total lesion measures 3–4 inches in diameter. The trypanosomal skin lesions may be located on the head or frequently on the legs and are usually accompanied by regional lymphadenopathy. The nodules subside spontaneously in about two weeks, often with no visible trace. In endemic areas few patients give a positive history of trypanosomal nodule, but it has

been reported by 70% of Europeans infected in Rhodesia. In addition, 91% of volunteers showed the typical lesions when infected experimentally.

Systemic manifestations occur two weeks after infection, concomitant with the invasion of the bloodstream by the trypanosomes. High fever, headache, and perhaps rigors are the initial manifestations of this stage of infection. Generalized enlargement of the lymph glands is very common; in the gambian disease the glands most characteristically enlarged are those in the posterior cervical triangle. In addition, six to eight weeks after the onset of illness, Caucasians sometimes develop a skin rash consisting of large, erythematous, circinate patches most evident on the chest and back. Neurological manifestations at this stage are nonspecific, consisting of severe headache, insomnia, inability to concentrate, delayed pain sensation, and, very rarely, delayed deep hyperesthesia (most marked over the tibia). The main laboratory findings in the acute stage of the infection are anemia, monocytosis, and markedly elevated serum levels of IgM.

(2) Subacute rhodesian trypanosomiasis. The course of the acute trypanosomiases varies with the causative organism. In the rhodesian form, the central nervous system is invaded within three to six weeks. This invasion is accompanied by recurrent bouts of fever, weakness, and constant headache, with signs of acute toxemia. At this stage, however, tachycardia is often seen, and death is due mainly to myocarditis. If the patient survives the first few weeks, weakness becomes more pronounced, anemia is marked, and there is often peripheral edema. Irritability, insomnia, and personality or mood changes develop. Somnolence is rare but mental slowness is frequent, and, if the patient is untreated, death from secondary infection or cardiac failure occurs within six to nine months.

(3) Chronic gambian trypanosomiasis. In the gambian form of infection, the blood-lymphatic stage may last for months, or sometimes years, before the typical signs of central nervous system involvement known as sleeping sickness occur. Involvement of the central nervous system in trypanosomiasis gambiense results in a form of meningoencephalomyelitis, with predominant involvement in the base of the brain. Before the days of specific treatment, analysis of 66 reported cases showed that drowsiness and an uncontrollable urge to sleep were present in 34% of the cases at the time of diagnosis and in all patients during the terminal stage of the infection. In addition, ex-

trapyramidal signs of tremors, rigidity, and ataxia were observed. Furthermore, 38% of these patients developed psychotic changes [4]. Prior to the use of specific therapy, the disease was invariably fatal; death usually resulted from malnutrition and intercurrent infection. It has also been demonstrated recently that patients with the gambian form of the disease are immunosuppressed, a state that may explain their increased susceptibility to secondary infections [5].

Diagnosis

The accompanying diagram illustrates the steps in the diagnosis of the African trypanosomiases (figure 1). Symptoms and signs suggestive of the disease necessitate a detailed geographic history since the infection is transmitted only in relatively limited areas. A visit to the major urban areas of East Africa is unlikely to result in exposure to *T. brucei rhodesiense,* but a game park safari provides an opportunity to acquire the infection. Similarly, only contact with tsetse flies in endemic foci in the rural areas of Central and West Africa suggests the possibility of gambian infection.

Tsetse flies are conspicuous insects about $\frac{1}{2}$ inch long and brown to grey in color. When they are at rest, the proboscis characteristically projects beyond the head, and the wings are folded one over the other. As tsetse bites are painful, contact with the flies is usually recollected. Nevertheless, a symptomatic individual with a positive geographic history requires a thorough search for trypanosomes. Such a search can be accomplished most easily by preparation of a thick blood smear. A small drop of blood is placed in the center of a slide and is spread out with a corner of another slide to cover an area about three to four times larger. Examination of fresh smears will demonstrate motile, active organisms; dried smears are stained for 30 min with Giemsa stain (Fisher Scientific, Fairlawn, N.J.). If the thick smear is negative, a simple concentration method should be used. Heparinized blood (10 ml) is lysed by the addition of 30 ml of 0.87% NH_4Cl (870 mg of NH_4Cl in 100 ml of water) and centrifuged at 1,000 g (about 2,000 rpm) for 15 min; the sediment is then examined or stained in the same manner as the blood smears. Material for examination can also be obtained by aspiration of enlarged lymph nodes. Since invasion of the central nervous system is an ever-present danger, a sample of the cerebrospinal fluid

must be drawn and centrifuged at 1,000 g for 15 min; the sediment should then be examined for the organisms as described above. Continued failure to demonstrate trypanosomes may necessitate the ip inoculation of 1 ml of the patient's blood into two rats and examination of their blood for the parasites two weeks later. This method is of value only when *T.b. rhodesiense* infection is suspected.

Management

Effective but toxic therapeutic agents are available for treatment of the African trypanosomiases [3, 6]. Suramin (antrypol; available from the Parasitic Drug Service of the Center for Disease Control, Atlanta, Ga.) is the drug of choice for treatment of the bloodstream stages of both types of trypanosome infection. A test dose of 100 mg is given iv for detection of the rare idiosyncratic patients who may suffer from shock and collapse. One gram is then given iv on days 1, 3, 7, 14, and 21. Toxic reactions to suramin include pruritis, papular eruptions, and, most important, some degree of damage to the kidneys. The urine should be tested before each injection. Although mild albuminuria is no indication for the suspension of therapy, in the presence of marked proteinuria, casts, or red cells, suramin administration should be stopped. If the patient has central nervous system involvement, therapy should be continued with melarsoprol as outlined below. Otherwise, the bloodstream stages can be cleared with a course of 10 daily im injections of pentamidine 3-mg base/kg of body weight (obtained from the Parasitic Drug Service, Center for Disease Control).

Involvement of the central nervous system requires the use of melarsoprol, an arsenical compound that crosses the blood-brain barrier (Parasitic Drug Service, Center for Disease Control). Therapy with this drug should commence after the first week of suramin administration. Melarsoprol is administered iv in doses of 1.5, 2.0, and 2.2 mg/kg of body weight at 48-hr intervals. One week later, doses of 2.5, 3.0, and 3.6 mg/kg are injected on a similar schedule; finally, after another interval of a week, there is a third course of three injections, each of 3.6 mg/kg of body weight. Patients receiving melarsoprol should be monitored closely for the toxic effects of arsenic, the most serious being encephalopathy and exfoliative dermatitis.

Chemoprophylaxis of trypanosomiasis gambiense with pentamidine has been introduced for the control

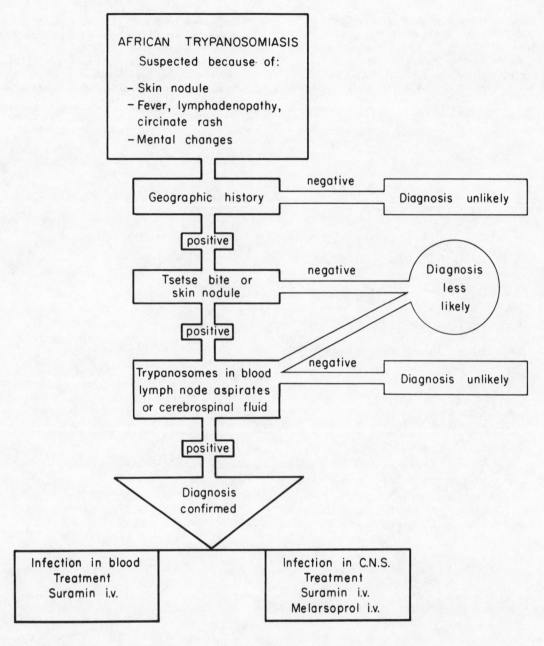

Figure 1. Progression to a definitive diagnosis of African trypanosomiasis. C.N.S. = central nervous system.

of disease in individuals, small groups, or whole communities in West Africa. However, the general consensus is that prophylaxis is not advisable for visitors to the endemic areas; reliance should be placed on rapid diagnosis and treatment if infection should occur.

References

1. Baker, J. R. Epidemiology of African sleeping sickness. *In* Ciba Foundation Symposium 20 (new series). Associated Scientific Publishers, Amsterdam, 1974, p. 29–50.
2. Spencer, H. S., Gibson, J. J., Brodsky, R. E., Schultz, M. G.

Imported African trypanosomiasis in the United States. Ann. Intern. Med. 82:633–638, 1975.

3. Mulligan, H. W. [ed.]. The African trypanosomiases. John Wiley and Sons, New York, 1970. 950 p.

4. Duggan, A. J., Hutchinson, M. P. Sleeping sickness in Europeans: a review of 109 cases. J. Trop. Med. Hyg. 69:124–131, 1966.

5. Greenwood, B. M., Whittle, H. C., Molyneux, D. H. Immunosuppression in gambian trypanosomiasis. Trans. R. Soc. Trop. Med. Hyg. 67:846–850, 1970.

6. Apted, F. I. C. Trypanosomiasis (African). *In* B. G. Maegraith and H. M. Gilles [ed.]. Management and treatment of tropical diseases. Blackwell Scientific Publications, Oxford and Edinburgh, 1971, p. 533–549.

American Trypanosomiasis

Trypanosomiasis cruzi, or Chagas' disease, occurs only in the western hemisphere; thus it has come to be known as American trypanosomiasis. This insect-transmitted protozoan infection is considered to be one of the major health problems of South America, largely because it is essentially untreatable [1]. It is particularly prevalent in Brazil, Argentina, Uruguay, Chile, and Venezuela but also occurs in Central America and in the Caribbean. In 1960 the World Health Organization estimated that there were seven million infected individuals and 30 million persons at risk.

The causative organism, *Trypanosoma cruzi,* infects both wild and domestic animals in addition to humans and is transmitted by a group of blood-sucking insects known as *Reduvid* bugs. In the United States these insect vectors have been found in all southeastern states as far north as Maryland [2], and infection has been reported in some mammalian species. Infection of humans, however, appears to be very rare; only two autochthonous cases of Chagas' disease have been reported. Thus, cases encountered in the United States would most probably be in immigrants or travelers from endemic areas.

Life Cycle

During its passage between vertebrate and insect hosts, *Trypansoma cruzi* undergoes several major morphologic changes [3]. The hematophagous insect vector, which belongs to the family Reduviidae, ingests the parasite in the blood of man and other mammalian species. The organisms pass to the midgut of the insects, transform into amastigotes (without a flagellum), and multiply; by six to 30 days the infective metacyclic forms appear in the rectum of the insects. The insect vectors often defecate while having their blood meal. The infective stage of the trypanosomes is passed in the feces, and although its mode of entry into the host is unclear, it is reportedly capable of penetrating intact skin or mucous membranes. In 14–28 days the trypomastigotes can be detected in the peripheral blood. They are 16–20 μm long with a pointed posterior end, a curved stumpy body (typically C-shaped in stained smears), and a flagellum that lies in the outer border of an undulating membrane and extends anteriorly beyond the body. Within a few weeks the trypomastigotes invade the reticuloendothelial system, the striated muscles, and the cardiac musculature and transform into amastigotes, which are rounded organisms 1.5–4.0 μm in diameter. These forms multiply by binary fission, forming nest-like cysts that destroy the host cells. Some of the parasites revert to the trypomastigote stage and reenter the bloodstream, where they may be ingested by the blood-sucking insects.

Epidemiology

Infection of humans with *T. cruzi* has been reported only in the western hemisphere and is prevalent primarily in the rural areas of South America, where the socioeconomic status of the people is low. Houses built of adobe, mud, or cane with numerous cracks in the walls provide the necessary habitat and breeding place for the insect vector in close proximity to man. Additional important factors in the epidemiology of Chagas' disease are the degree of adaptation of the Reduviidae to human habitation, the prevalence of infection in animal reservoirs, and the virulence of different strains of the parasite. In addition, transmission of *T. cruzi* by blood transfusion is a major danger in endemic areas and may occur in nonendemic areas as well. Infection has also been transmitted by contaminated syringes, in laboratory accidents, and through the placenta. A recent paper from Argentina described reactivation of *T. cruzi* infection in two leukemic patients treated with antimetabolites.

in several mammalian species that are widespread in the western hemisphere. The most important wild-reservoir hosts in the United States are opossums and raccoons, with infection rates of 17% and 2%, respectively. The prevalence of infection in reduvids has been estimated at 40%–60% in the endemic regions of South America and at 20%–25% in Mexico and the southwestern United States. In the southeastern states the insect vectors are rare, but *T. cruzi* infection is common in the opossum. Serologic evidence for human infection has been found in southern Texas;

1.8% of 500 unselected individuals and 2.5% of 117 persons who had been bitten by the insects had significant titers of antibody. In contrast, none of almost 4,000 sera from southern Georgia contained antibody. The rarity of infection in humans in the United States may be due to relatively low virulence of the strains of *T. cruzi* involved, zoophilia of the insect vectors, and better housing conditions of the human hosts.

Disease Syndromes

The initial infection is usually occult but may be manifested in an acute form; this acute illness is rarely seen, even in endemic areas, and subsides spontaneously in 90%–95% of cases within one to four months. The infection then remains asymptomatic for periods of as long as several decades, after which some individuals gradually begin to show the chronic manifestations of the disease. It has been estimated that, over a period of 24 years, approximately 10% of all serologically positive individuals develop clinically overt chronic forms of Chagas' disease.

(1) Acute trypanosomiasis. This form of the disease usually occurs in childhood in endemic areas and will probably not be seen by physicians in the United States; however, it is worth mentioning since it provides a historical basis for diagnosis of the chronic forms. In one recent report, a quarter of infected individuals had no reaction at the site of entry of the trypanosomes, 50% developed a lesion on the face (unilateral painless palpebral swelling—Romaña's sign), while 25% had a nodular lesion on the body (chagoma). Both types of lesion are accompanied by enlargement of the draining lymph nodes. It should be noted, however, that manifestations of acute trypanosomiasis vary from one endemic area to another and may be altogether absent. The lesions are thought to be due to multiplication of the parasite, but some evidence indicates that local edema can be produced by feces of uninfected insects in sensitized individuals. General dissemination of the parasites via the bloodstream may result in malaise, fever, muscular pain, nontender lymphadenopathy, and hepatosplenomegaly. Some degree of cardiac involvement occurs in every overt case, with tachycardia and triple rhythm; abnormalities are found in electrocardiograms of 43% of these patients. The death rate in acute trypanosomiasis has been estimated at 10% and is related either to heart failure or meningoencephalitis.

(2) Chronic trypanosomiasis. The pathogenesis of chronic Chagas' disease is related to the destruction of autonomic ganglia and/or myositis. Marked denervation of the heart, esophagus, colon, bronchi, and other hollow viscera has been reported. Neither the mechanism of destruction of ganglion cells nor the time of the destruction is known [4]. With respect to myositis, recent evidence suggests that cell-mediated autoimmune reactions may play in important role in destruction of myocardial cells.

(a) Cardiomyopathy. In endemic areas cardiomyopathy of trypanosomiasis is the leading cause of both cardiac disease and sudden death. Patients commonly present with symptoms and signs of congestive heart failure and have a grossly enlarged heart. Chronic lymphocytic myocarditis is the major pathological lesion. Signs of valvular damage and dysfunction, however, are exceedingly rare. Two-thirds of the patients have some disturbances of cardiac conduction with right bundle branch block occurring most frequently.

(b) Megaorgans. Megaesophagus and megacolon, conditions in which these hollow viscera are markedly enlarged and dilated, are by far the most common forms of digestive tract involvement in trypanosomiasis [5]. The prevalence of the megaorgans differs in the various endemic areas, but these conditions are particularly common in Brazil. The usual clinical presentation of megaesophagus is dysphagia and regurgitation, and that of megacolon is constipation. Megastomach, megaduodenum, megabronchus, megaureter, etc., have been reported but are quite rare.

Diagnosis

The sequence of steps necessary for the diagnosis of Chagas' disease is shown in figure 1. When a patient presents with suggestive symptoms or signs, a geographic history should be obtained, since Chagas' disease does not occur outside the western hemisphere and is endemic only in South America. If the geographic history is positive, it should then be ascertained whether the patient has lived under conditions in which the disease is transmitted to humans (e.g., mud huts) and whether he/she has a history of insect bites and their sequelae. The probable duration of infection should then be estimated, since the laboratory diagnosis of acute cases (first few weeks) differs from that of chronic cases. For acute cases both un-

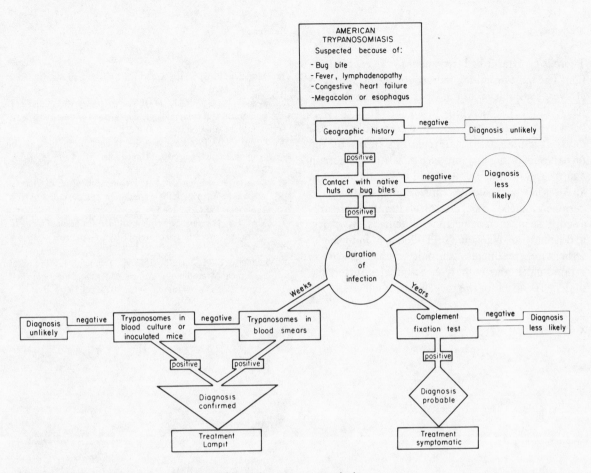

Figure 1. The progression to a diagnosis of American trypanosomiasis.

stained and Giemsa-stained fixed blood smears should be examined to demonstrate the motile trypomastigotes and the typical C-shaped stained organisms, respectively. Since concentration of the trypomastigotes can facilitate diagnosis in light infections, 10 ml of heparinized blood should be lysed by the addition of 30 ml of 0.87% NH_4Cl (870 mg of NH_4Cl in 100 ml of water) and centrifuged at 1,000 g (about 2,000 rpm) for 15 min; the pellet should be examined for trypanosomes. Continued failure to demonstrate the organisms necessitates: *(1)* culture of blood on diphasic blood-agar medium (NIH method) [6] in screw-capped culture tubes incubated at room temperature and examined every two weeks for three months; *(2)* ip injection of 1 ml of the patient's blood into two albino mice and examination of the mouse blood for the parasites every week for one month; and *(3)* xenodiagnosis, or allowing laboratory-reared reduvids to feed on the patient and examining the rectal contents of the vector 30–60 days later. The third

technique is the most sensitive diagnostic method but is essentially unavailable in the United States.

Demonstration of the trypanosomes by any of the above-mentioned techniques establishes the diagnosis. If the patient has been infected for longer than a few weeks, however, it is unlikely that a definitive diagnosis can be made by blood examination. Xenodiagnosis is the only technique that may provide an answer in chronic *T. cruzi* infections. The typical clinical presentation, geographic history, and report of insects in the household are criteria of major importance at this stage. In addition, a complement fixation test (available at the Center for Disease Control, Atlanta, Ga.) is helpful. Unfrozen serum samples (1–2 ml) should be mailed to state laboratories, from which they will be forwarded to the Center for Disease Control. It has been estimated that this test yields positive results in 80% of patients with chronic Chagas' heart disease and in 90% of those with megaesophagus.

Management

There is no established treatment for *T. cruzi* infection. The most promising therapeutic agent, Lampit,® (Bayer; available from the Center for Disease Control, Atlanta, Ga.) is a nitrofuran derivative that has been used in regimens of 5–15 mg/kg daily for 120 days. It eliminates the circulating forms of the trypanosomes and may produce parasitologic cure in acute cases. Therefore, it should be administered in all cases in which parasites can be demonstrated in the peripheral blood. Side effects of Lampit® are frequently seen, such as peripheral neuritis, psychosis and hemolytic anemia in G6PD-deficient individuals. Otherwise, treatment of chronic Chagas' disease is symptomatic and palliative. Surgical interference may be required for the megaorgan syndromes.

References

1. Marsden, P. D. South American trypanosomiasis. Int. Rev. Trop. Med. 4:97–121, 1971.
2. Woody, N. C., Woody, H. B. American trypanosomiasis. I. Clinical and epidemiologic background of Chagas' disease in the United States. J. Pediatr. 58:568–580, 1961.
3. Levine, N. D. Protozoan parasites of domestic animals and of man. 2nd ed. Burgess, Minneapolis, Minn., 1973, p. 54–58.
4. Anselmi, A., Moleiro, F. Pathogenic mechanisms in Chagas' cardiomyopathy. Ciba Foundation Symposium 20 (New Series), 1974, p. 125–136.
5. Alva, J. J. The gastroenterological manifestation of Chagas' disease. Acta Gastroenterol. Latin America 4:33–43, 1972.
6. Lennette, E. H., Spaulding, E. H., Truant, J. P. Manual of Clinical Microbiology. 2nd ed. American Society for Microbiology, Washington, D.C., 1974, p. 616.

Ascariasis and Toxocariasis

Ascariasis

Ascaris lumbricoides, also known as the "giant intestinal round worm," has been known since ancient times because of its foot-long size and its great prevalence. In 1947 it was estimated that there were 644 million people, or approximately one-quarter of the world's population, with ascariasis. Since this ubiquitous parasite is difficult to control and there has been considerable population growth in the last 30 years, it can now be estimated that *A. lumbricoides* infects one billion people. In the United States, a recent review suggested that four million people, mainly in the southeastern section, have ascariasis [1].

Enormous egg output by the worms and resistance of the eggs to the external environment facilitate the spread of infection. The usual mode of transmission of ascariasis is by ingestion of fecally contaminated raw vegetables and fruits. As with other worm infections, *Ascaris* do not multiply in man, and disease is usually related to intensity of infection. Fortunately, ascariasis appears to be asymptomatic in the vast majority of cases, but even a small proportion of individuals with disease manifestations would constitute an enormous burden on mankind.

Life cycle. Adult *A. lumbricoides* are large, pinkish-white nematodes (males, 15–30 cm × 3 mm; females, 25–35 cm × 4 mm) with three fleshy lips at the anterior end and an attenuated posterior end. The normal habitat of these worms is the lumen of the small intestine. Each female produces approximately 200,000 eggs per day over a life span of about one year. The fertilized eggs (60 × 40 μm) have an outer albuminoid layer, a thick transparent shell, and inner membranes which are highly impermeable. The eggs are passed in the feces in an unembryonated state, and under suitable conditions mature into infective larvae in approximately three weeks. When fully embryonated eggs are swallowed, the larvae (250 × 15 μm) hatch, penetrate the wall of the small intestine, and pass into the circulation within which they are carried into the lungs. After several days they break out of the blood vessels into the alveoli and pass up through the respiratory tract to the esophagus where they are swallowed. When the larvae arrive in the small intestine again, they develop into adult male or female worms and begin production of eggs. The time elapsed from ingestion of eggs to production of eggs by adults is approximately two months.

Epidemiology. The great success of *A. lumbricoides* as a parasite of man is based on an extremely high output of eggs and on their great resistance to the external environment. Under optimal conditions of warmth and moisture, the eggs embryonate within two weeks, and they remain infective for months. Infection is continuous during the year in warm moist climates but is seasonal in dry areas, occurring only in the rainy season. The prevalence and intensity of ascariasis is highest in children, particularly those with frequent contact with soil. The infection is also spread by fecally contaminated fruits and vegetables and can be transferred to foodstuffs by flies. *Ascaris suum,* the common ascarid of the pig, is similar morphologically to *A. lumbricoides* but can be distinguished from the human parasite; studies in volunteers have shown that it is far less infective to man than is *A. lumbricoides.*

Since the worms do not multiply in man, different levels of infection are seen in endemic areas, with most individuals having light to moderate worm burdens. In a survey in Colombia, 72% of infected individuals had light infections (less than one to 19 eggs/mg of feces), and only 5% had heavy infections (> 200 eggs/mg of feces) [2]. Intensity of infection is probably related largely to degree of exposure. In endemic areas, many studies have revealed a rapid rate of reinfection after treatment, as most individuals are infected again within eight to 10 months. Since the life span of the worm is relatively short, a steady state is probably reached that is related to the input of new worms and the death of old ones.

Disease syndromes. Ascariasis may well be the most prevalent single infection of man. As the majority of infections are of low intensity, overt disease is relatively rare in ascariasis. Children have the highest prevalence and intensity of *A. lumbricoides* infection, however, and the various disease syndromes are seen most frequently in the younger age groups. The more common problems are possible impairment of nutritional status, intestinal and biliary obstruction, and, where exposure is intermittent, seasonal pneumonitis.

In a careful study of nutritional balance performed in India, children with moderately heavy infections were shown to have mild to moderate impairment of digestion and absorption of dietary protein [3]. In Colombia, children with heavy infections, averaging 48–95 worms, had a 7.2% impairment in dietary nitrogen absorption, and two-thirds of the children studied had a moderate steatorrhea involving 13.4% of dietary fat [4]. It has been suggested, therefore, that children with large parasite loads and low protein intake might suffer from significant nutritional impairment. However, a controlled study of the nutritional status of children with moderate to heavy *Ascaris* infections and "far from optimal" dietary conditions performed in the southern United States has revealed no significant differences between uninfected and infected children with respect to anthropometric measurements and few significant differences on physical examination and in laboratory tests [5].

Intestinal obstruction is one of the serious consequences of ascariasis [6, 7]. It is usually due to a mass of worms obstructing the lumen of the small bowel and is found largely in young children (peak incidence in children aged one to six years) with very heavy infections [7]. The major symptoms and signs are vomiting, abdominal distention, and abdominal pain. The patient may pass worms in vomitus and stools during the attack.

Biliary obstruction with *A. lumbricoides* has been reported in particularly large numbers from China and the Philippines [8]. It has been suggested that the likelihood of bile duct invasion is increased in heavier infections. In a pediatric study, biliary obstruction tended to occur more frequently in older children. It is also seen in adults. Major signs and symptoms are colicky epigastric pain in almost all cases, nausea and vomiting in 30%–80% of cases, and fever in similar percentages of cases; as this is an acute syndrome, jaundice is rare.

With respect to pulmonary manifestations, *Ascaris* antigens are highly allergenic, and it has been suggested that this helminthic infection is a major cause of asthma. There is, however, little good evidence supporting this point of view. In fact, it is quite remarkable, considering the allergenicity of the organism and the migration of the larvae through the lungs, that there is so little pulmonary disease directly attributable to *A. lumbricoides* in highly endemic areas. In 13,000 patients with moderate to heavy infections in Colombia, only four cases were found of a Loeffler's pneumonia-like syndrome involving acute

respiratory symptoms, transient pulmonary infiltrates, and peripheral eosinophilia [2]. This syndrome, however, has been reported with relative frequency in Saudi Arabia and other countries where ascariasis occurs only seasonally and has been found largely in adults [9].

The literature on ascariasis is replete with unusual case reports and autopsy findings, but this is not surprising in view of the great prevalence of this infection.

Diagnosis. The progression to a diagnosis of ascariasis is shown in figure 1. A significant degree of infection accompanied by disease manifestations is most likely to be seen in young children from tropical and subtropical countries. In the United States, the majority of such patients will come from the southeastern states or Puerto Rico. Intermittent or unusual exposures may lead to the development of an eosinophilic pneumonia, which may be seen in adults. A positive geographic history should be followed by careful questioning about contact with soil (young children) and ingestion of raw, nonpeelable vegetables and fruit. A stool examination should follow.

Since a female *A. lumbricoides* worm produces an average of 200,000 eggs per day, there is no difficulty in finding eggs in the stool [10]. Thus a concentration technique is not necessary, and stools can be examined by direct smear. A drop of saline is placed on a microscope slide, a small portion of feces is emulsified in it, and a cover slip is placed on top. The density of the preparation should be such that fine print can be read through the smear. These preparations usually contain 1.0–1.5 mg of feces, and the egg count is multiplied by 750 to estimate the number of eggs per g of feces. This technique should suffice to detect the presence of a single female worm.

Diagnosis of intestinal and biliary obstruction is usually made on a high index of suspicion plus evidence of past or present infection with *Ascaris*. Seasonal pneumonia is particularly suggested by a high eosinophilia.

Management. Of the several drugs available for treatment of ascariasis, the piperazine compounds are the most versatile. For uncomplicated cases, piperazine citrate (Antepar®; Burroughs Wellcome Co., Research Triangle Park, N.C.) is administered orally in a single daily dose of 50 mg/kg (maximal dose, 3.5 g) for two days. As this drug narcotizes the worms, it is also efficacious in the treatment of the intestinal obstruction syndrome. Most of these cases should be treated conservatively with parenteral fluids, intu-

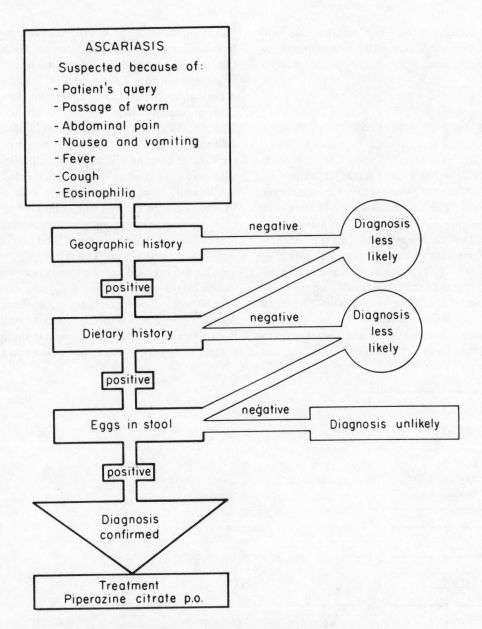

Figure 1. The progression to the diagnosis and treatment of ascariasis; p.o. = perorally.

bation and decompression, and instillation of piperazine syrup in an initial dose of 150 mg/kg (maximum, 3 g) followed with six doses of 65 mg/kg (maximum, 1 g) at 12-hr intervals. The drug can also be used to treat biliary obstruction with an initial dose of 150 mg/kg followed by two doses of 65 mg/kg at 12-hr intervals. Only a relatively small proportion of cases have required surgical treatment: <20% in the case of intestinal obstruction and 5% in the case of biliary obstruction.

An alternative to the piperazine compounds for treating uncomplicated ascariasis is the broad spectrum anthelmintic, mebendazole (Vermox,® Ortho Pharmaceutical Corp., Raritan, N.J.), which is also effective for hookworm infection, trichuriasis, and enterobiasis. The recommended dose is 100 mg orally twice a day for 3 days regardless of body weight.

Pulmonary ascariasis is a self-limited disease which usually subsides in less than two weeks. General measures to alleviate respiratory difficulties and cough should be instituted, when indicated. Standard treatment for intestinal ascariasis can be administered after the worms develop to maturity in the small intestine.

Toxocariasis

Toxocariasis, also known as visceral larva migrans, is an infection of very young children by the canine or feline ascarids, *Toxocara canis* or *Toxocara cati,* which are worldwide in distribution [11]. In the natural canine host, patent egg producing intestinal infections are most common in puppies. Although dogs may be infected by ingestion of eggs, even more important is prenatal infection in which immature larvae in the tissues of the mother migrate into the fetus. Man, in whom the development of adult worms is extremely rare, is infected by the oral route. Only very young children (between the ages of one and four

years) appear to be susceptible to infection. In these hosts the immature larvae continue to migrate within the tissues, largely of the liver and lungs, for years. Epidemiologically, *T. canis* and *T. cati* are highly prevalent in dogs and cats throughout the world. A study in Britain revealed eggs of *Toxocara* species in 24% of 800 soil samples taken from public places [12]. Infection appears to be most common in children with the habit of pica and is also more prevalent in children who have close contact with dogs and cats.

Clinically, visceral larva migrans is characterized by fever, hepatomegaly (87%), pulmonary symptoms (50%) including coughing, wheezing, and X-ray evidence of pulmonary infiltration, and marked eosinophilia (virtually 100%). The severity of the disease appears to be related to the intensity of infection, but visceral larva migrans is generally a benign entity, with 97% of symptomatic patients showing complete recovery over a period of years. *Toxocara* have also been reported in many other organs, the most important being the eye where the involvement is usually

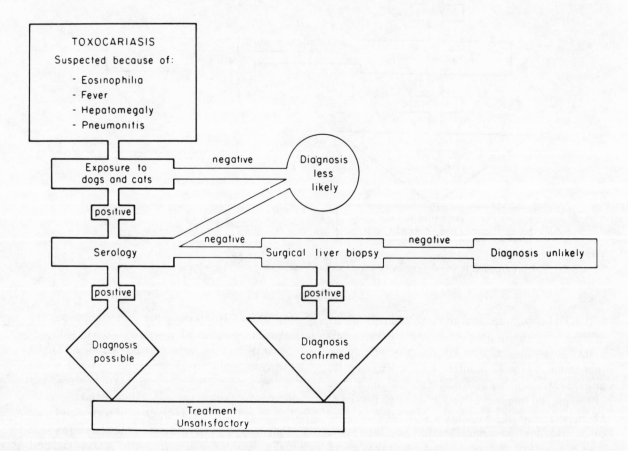

Figure 2.   The progression to the diagnosis and treatment of toxocariasis.

unilateral and is seen in older children. Cerebral and myocardial symptoms are occasionally observed.

The progression to a diagnosis of toxocariasis is shown in figure 2. Known exposure to dogs and cats is important, but its absence does not rule out this infection. The diagnosis is suggested by positive serological tests using *Toxocara* and *Ascaris* antigens. For serological testing, 1 ml of serum should be sent at ambient temperature to state health laboratories to be forwarded to the Center for Disease Control, Atlanta, Ga. 30333. A definitive diagnosis can be achieved only by open, wedge liver biopsy with the preparation of serial sections; these sections should be examined by an expert in the identification of the larval organisms. No significantly effective treatment is available for visceral larva migrans, but the disease almost invariably subsides. Highly symptomatic cases may benefit from treatment with corticosteroids. Prevention is best achieved by limiting contact of very young children with dogs and cats, discouraging pica, and making sure that these animals are adequately dewormed.

References

1. Warren, K. S. Helminthic diseases endemic in the United States. Am. J. Trop. Med. Hyg. 23:723–730, 1974.

2. Spillman, R. K. Pulmonary ascariasis in tropical communities. Am. J. Trop. Med. Hyg. 24:791–800, 1975.

3. Venkatachalam, P. S., Patwardhan, V. N. The role of *Ascaris lumbricoides* in the nutrition of the host: effect of ascariasis on digestion of protein. Trans. R. Soc. Trop. Med. Hyg. 47:169–175, 1953.

4. Tripathy, K., Gonzales, F., Lotero, H., Bolaños, O. Effects of *Ascaris* infection on human nutrition. Am. J. Trop. Med. Hyg. 20:212–218, 1971.

5. Blumenthal, D. S., Schultz, M. G. Effects of *Ascaris* infection on nutritional status in children. Am. J. Trop. Med. Hyg. 25:682–690, 1976.

6. Blumenthal, D. S., Schultz, M. G. Incidence of intestinal obstruction in children infected with *Ascaris lumbricoides*. Am. J. Trop. Med. Hyg. 24:801–805, 1975.

7. Louw, J. H. Abdominal complications of *Ascaris lumbricoides* infestation in children. Br. J. Surg. 53:510–521, 1966.

8. Chin-Che, C., Cheng-Teh, H. Biliary ascariasis in childhood. A clinical analysis of 788 cases. Chin. Med. J. 85:167–171, 1966.

9. Gelpi, A. P., Mustafa, A. Ascaris pneumonia. Am. J. Med. 44:377–389, 1968.

10. Melvin, D. M., Brooke, M. M. Laboratory procedures for the diagnosis of intestinal parasites. Publication no. (CDC) 75–8282. Center for Disease Control, Atlanta, 1974, p. 37–38, 165.

11. Mok, C. H. Visceral larva migrans. A discussion based on review of the literature. Clin. Pediatr. 7:565–573, 1968.

12. Borg, O. A., Woodruff, A. W. Prevalence of infective ova of *Toxocara* species in public places. Br. Med. J. 4:470–472, 1973.

Echinococcosis

Echinococcosis (hydatid disease) in humans is caused by the larval stage of the canine tapeworm *Echinococcus granulosus.* The infection is a zoonosis, with man being an incidental host to the natural cycle of transmission between carnivores and various herbivorous animals.

Human infection is characterized by space-occupying hydatid cysts found mostly in the liver and lungs but also in other organs. Man is an intermediate host for *E. granulosus,* and the growing cysts contain multiplying larvae; this parasite is therefore one of the few helminths that replicate within the human body. The adult tapeworms are found in canines, usually dogs and wolves.

E. granulosus is worldwide in distribution but is most frequently found in the sheep- and cattle-raising areas of Australasia, South America, South Africa, the Soviet Union, and the Mediterranean littoral. The infection is relatively uncommon in the United States, but both imported and autochthonous cases have been reported. Indigenously acquired cases have been described in 15 states, and the complete cycle of transmission involving sheep, dogs, and humans has been found in California and Utah [1]. Echinococcosis is also endemic in Alaska but has a different epidemiological pattern [2].

Life Cycle

The adult *Echinococcus,* found in the small intestine of dogs and wolves, is a small tapeworm 3–6 mm long, consisting of a head (scolex) armed with hooklets and suckers, a neck, and three segments. Rupture of the terminal gravid segment releases up to 500 eggs, which are discharged in the feces.

On ingestion by intermediate hosts such as sheep or humans, the embryos escape from the eggs in the duodenum, penetrate the mucosa, and pass via the portal veins to the liver, where most of them are trapped. Those that pass through the liver are usually arrested in the lungs, but some embryos may reach the systemic circulation, where they may seed any organ. Wherever the parasites lodge, they either are destroyed by an inflammatory reaction or develop into hydatid cysts. The embryo undergoes central vesiculation, increases in size, and differentiates into an outer laminated membrane and an inner germinal layer. From this inner layer buds develop, which again vesiculate to form brood capsules. Larval scolices (rudimentary heads) arise on the inner surface of the brood capsule by further internal budding and may be released into the hydatid fluid if the brood capsule ruptures. Sometimes the brood capsules develop an outer laminated layer, thus becoming daughter cysts within the parent cyst. The mature hydatid cyst, which is usually spherical, grows slowly over many years and may reach 20 cm in diameter. When bones are involved, the dense tissues do not permit the parasite to assume its normal spherical shape, the fibrous capsule is absent and naked excrescences penetrate the bone cavities to form multiple outpouchings containing little fluid.

After the death of the intermediate host, the larval hydatid may be eaten by a dog or another definitive host, whereupon the released scolices attach to the small intestinal mucosa and mature into multiple adult worms over a period of six to eight weeks.

Epidemiology

The prevalence of human echinococcosis is dependent upon the association of man with infected canines. There are two epidemiological patterns, domestic and sylvatic, in both of which members of the canine family are the definitive hosts of the adult worms. The more important cycle is adapted to domesticated dogs, which are infected when they eat the contaminated viscera of sheep, cattle, or pigs; the cycle of transmission continues when the eggs passed in the dogs' feces are eaten by the herbivorous intermediate hosts. Echinococcosis is most frequently reported in regions of the world where livestock is a major industry. It is especially common in the sheep-raising areas where dogs are fed uncooked offal. Surveys in several parts of the United States, including California, Utah, and Mississippi, have revealed that 1%–5% of sheep, cattle, and pigs are infected with *E. granulosus.* Man is infected most frequently by direct contact with infected dogs but also by ingestion of contaminated soil, vegetables, or water.

A sylvatic epidemiological cycle is seen in the zones of tundra and northern coniferous forest of Alaska and Canada, where a strain which has sometimes been called *E. granulosus* var. *canadensis* also occurs. The adult form is found in the wolf, and the larval stage is adapted to large deer such as moose, reindeer, and caribou.

Disease Syndromes

The majority of infections with *E. granulosus* are asymptomatic. Many infections are detected during a routine chest X ray, during the investigation of an unrelated condition, or at autopsy. Since almost any organ can be invaded, the symptoms and signs which may be encountered are protean. The anatomical distribution of cysts may vary with geographical area, but an indication is given by the following distribution of 1,802 cysts recorded in the Australasian Hyadatid Registry: liver, 63%; lung, 25%; muscles, 5%; bone, 3%; kidney, 2%; spleen and brain, 1%; and heart, thyroid, breast, prostate, parotid, and pancreas, all <1%. Multiple cysts are found in approximately 20% of patients.

Patients with symptomatic infections usually present with the features of a space-occupying lesion. Since the liver is a large organ of uniform function in a distensible area of the body, hepatic cysts usually become quite large before producing symptoms, unless they are located in a strategic site such as the porta hepatis. Some patients may complain of abdominal discomfort or epigastric pain; others may have enlargement of the liver, especially of the right lobe. Many cysts, however, are revealed only by calcification seen on an abdominal radiograph. In view of the years required for symptoms to appear or calcification to develop, hepatic hydatids are seen most frequently in middle-aged or elderly patients.

Pulmonary hydatids are often found in children and younger patients. This fact may be accounted for in part by early discovery of this form in chest X rays for unrelated conditions or during mass surveys. Symptomatic patients may complain of hemoptysis, cough, or dyspnea. Intracranial cysts are likely to be symptomatic early in their development, presenting with the features of a slowly expanding space-occupying lesion. Hydatid disease of bone is often revealed by a spontaneous fracture, while hematuria or loin pain may be the first signs of a renal cyst.

The most important complications of hydatid cysts are rupture or infection. A leaking cyst may give rise to urticaria or precipitate an anaphylactic reaction. Furthermore, dissemination of scolices may lead to the establishment of secondary hydatid infections elsewhere in the body. Bacterial infection of a cyst resembles an abscess of the liver, lung, or other organ.

Diagnosis

An algorithm for the diagnosis and management of echinococcosis is given in figure 1. The infection may be suspected in an otherwise asymptomatic patient who is found by chance (on routine radiography) to have a lesion in the lungs or calcification in the liver area. Other patients may be noted to have hepatomegaly or may present with hemoptysis, fracture, urticaria, or any of a wide variety of symptoms and signs of a space-occupying lesion in any organ.

A geographic history must be taken. The diagnosis is more likely if the patient has lived in an area of the world where hydatid disease is prevalent. Inquiry should be made concerning intimate contact with dogs that may have been exposed to potentially infected offal. The disease is more likely, therefore, in people who have lived on sheep and cattle farms. There are unusual situations, however, such as in Wales, where infection occurs in small towns to which sheep have free access, and in Alaska, where dogs may impinge upon the sylvatic cycle by eating infected deer. Failure to obtain such a history does not exclude the diagnosis but renders it less likely.

All patients should have plain X rays of both the abdomen and the chest, since some have multiple cysts. The abdominal film may show a calcified round or oval cyst rim or spotty calcified densities, usually in the liver area. The chest film usually shows a round, uniformly dense lesion 1–20 cm in diameter, but calcification rarely occurs. There may be surrounding pneumonitis or atelectasis and, occasionally, a fluid level indicating rupture into a bronchus [3]. All patients with both hepatic and extrahepatic lesions should have a liver scan for detection of focal filling defects; cysts on the periphery of the liver often give an appearance of hepatic displacement. A suspicious liver defect may be further investigated by selective visceral angiography, which may demonstrate an avascular mass that is often surrounded by a characteristic halo of dye [4].

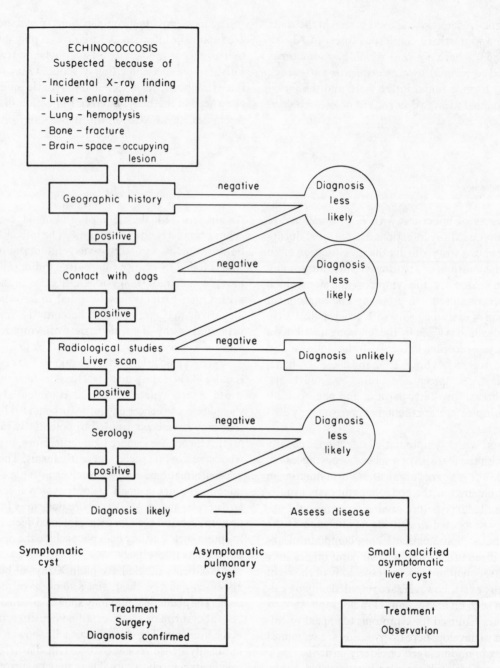

Figure 1. Progression to a definitive diagnosis of echinococcosis.

When a mass has been demonstrated, immunological tests may help in elucidating its hydatid nature. The Casoni skin test is not reliable, since it has not been standardized and false-positive results are obtained in up to 40% of patients. Sera may be sent to the Mycology and Parasitology Section, Center for Disease Control, Atlanta, Georgia for serological testing. Indirect HA titers of ≥1:32, and bentonite flocculation titers of ≥1:5 are considered positive. Serological tests yield positive results in approximately 85% of patients with liver cysts but in only 40% of patients with pulmonary echinococcosis. False-positive results (usually with low titers) may be found in patients with cirrhosis or collagen diseases and in those with other helminthic infections, especially cysticercosis [5].

Eosinophilia is uncommon, and abnormal results in tests of liver function are neither prominent nor diagnostic. A presumptive diagnosis must be made, therefore, on the basis of probabilities. On no account should an attempt be made to make a parasitological diagnosis by percutaneous needle puncture of a cyst, since this procedure may cause leakage leading to anaphylaxis or spread of the lesions. In patients in whom surgical intervention is appropriate, the definitive diagnosis is made by demonstration of the parasite at surgery.

Management

When the diagnosis is considered probable, the disease must be assessed and the benefits and risks of surgical intervention weighed. Surgery is indicated in all symptomatic patients but carries with it a small risk of death and a moderate incidence of morbidity. If the patient is asymptomatic and the cyst has been discovered by chance, then the location of the lesion, the age and fitness of the patient, and the strain of parasite must be considered. A small ($\leq$5 cm in diameter), calcified liver hydatid in an asymptomatic patient requires only observation, especially if the serological tests are negative. It is generally agreed that pulmonary cysts warrant operation, even in the asymptomatic patient, to prevent rupture, infection, and the attendant complications. An exception may be made in the case of *E. granulosus* var. *canadensis,* since such patients do not seem to develop complications readily [2]. Many surgical techniques have been used, but, if possible, the cyst should be removed entirely. To prevent spillage and dissemination, the cyst is carefully isolated, as much of the fluid as possible is aspirated, an equal volume of aqueous iodine solution to make a final solution of 1% is injected and allowed to mix for several minutes, then all of the fluid is aspirated, and the cyst is excised. The iodine kills the scolices within 1 min and probably produces fewer complications than formalin, which has been used in the past. Corticosteroid and antihistamine therapy

may be necessary if an anaphylactic reaction occurs as a result of spillage during the operation. Details of the surgical techniques used in hepatic, pulmonary, and bony hydatid disease have been described elsewhere [6–8].

Infection with Echinococcus multilocularis.   E. multilocularis infections are usually found in Europe and in the northern latitudes of Asia and North America but have been reported elsewhere. The adult worm is found in foxes as well as in domestic cats and dogs, while the larval form is found principally in field rodents. When man is infected, there is an aggregation of innumerable small cysts that multiply by exogenous budding to produce the so-called malignant hydatid; hydatids are usually found in the liver, and the honeycomb lesions may be confused with a malignancy. The prognosis is grave, with portal hypertension and liver failure often developing. Treatment is by surgical excision, if possible.

References

1. Kahn, J. B., Spruance, C., Harbottle, J., Cannon, P., Schultz, M. G. Echinococcosis in Utah. Am. J. Trop. Med. Hyg. 21:185–188, 1972.
2. Wilson, J. F., Diddams, A. C., Rausch, R. L. Cystic hydatid disease in Alaska: a review of 101 autochthonous cases of *Echinococcus granulosus* infection. Am. Rev. Resp. Dis. 98:1–15, 1968.
3. Balikian, J. P., Mudarris, F. F. Hydatid disease of the lungs: a roentgenologic study of 50 cases. Am. J. Roentgenol. Radium Ther. Nucl. Med. 122:692–707, 1974.
4. Garti, I., Deutsch, V. The angiographic diagnosis of echinococcosis of the liver and spleen. Clin. Radiol. 22:466–471, 1971.
5. Kagan, I. G., Norman, L. Serodiagnosis of parasitic disease. *In* E. H. Lennette, E. H. Spaulding, and J. P. Truant [ed.]. Manual of clinical microbiology. 2nd ed. American Society for Microbiology, Washington, D.C., 1974, p. 645–647.
6. Hankins, J. R. Management of complicated hydatid cysts. Ann. Surg. 158:1020–1034, 1963.
7. Sarsam, A. Surgery of pulmonary hydatid cysts: review of 155 cases. J. Thorac. Cardiovasc. Surg. 62:663–668, 1971.
8. Booz, M. K. The management of hydatid disease of bone and joint. J. Bone Joint Surg. 54B:698–709, 1972.

Enterobiasis

Enterobiasis, or pinworm, is by far the most common of all helminthic infections in the United States, with an estimated 42 million cases [1]. The infection is worldwide in distribution and occurs most frequently in children (in both well-developed and developing countries). Pinworm is no respecter of socioeconomic status, but the infection tends to be more frequent under crowded institutional conditions. It is essentially a trivial, occult infection in which the major (although relatively infrequent) symptom is perianal pruritus. Granulomatous inflammatory lesions surrounding the worms, larvae, or eggs in the tissues of the abdominal viscera have been reported, but such lesions seem to be exceedingly rare, given the prevalence of enterobiasis. Probably the greatest problem associated with this helminthic parasite is the so-called "pinworm neurosis," bred of the fear and aversion with which these essentially harmless organisms are viewed. Although enterobiasis tends to recur despite rigorous cleanliness, the infection is easily treated and cured with nontoxic drugs.

Life Cycle

Enterobius vermicularis is a white thread-like worm 1 cm in length. Its simple life cycle begins at the mouth of the host with the ingestion of embryonated eggs, proceeds with the development of adult worms of both sexes in the intestinal lumen, and terminates two weeks to two months later, when dying, gravid female worms deposit their eggs in the perianal area [2]. The eggs embryonate within 6 hr and may be passed back to the mouth by a highly efficient mechanism: the worms or the eggs induce anal pruritus by means as yet unknown, and scratching leads to direct anus-finger-mouth transmission. The eggs also become widespread in the environment on clothing, bedding, and in house dust; some of them remain viable and infective for as long as 20 days. On ingestion, the embryos hatch in the duodenum, molt

twice, and develop to adult male or female worms 0.3 mm wide and 5 and 10 mm long, respectively. Their main habitat is the cecum and adjacent areas, including the appendix. The worms lie free in the intestinal lumen; there is little evidence that they penetrate into the tissues under normal conditions. After copulation in the cecal region, the gravid females migrate at night to the perianal and perineal area, where each lays 5,000–17,000 eggs and then dies.

Epidemiology

Man is the only natural host of *E. vermicularis*. Although primates are reported to have similar parasites, the strains that infect humans and animals are not intertransmissible. The most common means of infection appears to be the anus-hand-mouth system, but the eggs may be ubiquitous in the environment on clothing, bedclothes, and dust and may even be inhaled. The eggs become infective 6 hr after they are laid, and under proper conditions of temperature and humidity they may remain infective for 20 days.

E. vermicularis infection occurs in all socioeconomic groups throughout the world, but for yet unknown reasons enteriobiasis is less prevalent in black than in white people. The infection is common in all parts of the United States, including Alaska [1]. Enterobiasis is most frequent in children five through nine years old, but infection may be found among almost all age groups. Conservative overall estimates of prevalence are 30% in children and 16% in adults. The prevalence of infection may be extremely high (96%) in institutions [1]. Intensity of infection (as measured by worm counts after treatment) has revealed an average of 58 worms per four- through 10-year-old child compared with 16 worms per 11- through 16-year-old child [3].

Disease Syndrome

Perianal disease.   The great prevalence of enterobiasis illustrates well the difference between infection and disease in helminthic infections. Worm burdens have seldom been measured, and the relation of disease to intensity of infection remains unknown. Nevertheless, most symptomatic infections are found during the period when the prevalence and intensity of pinworm infection are maximal. In one careful hospital-based study in Boston of children from two to 12 years old, none of the signs and symptoms usually ascribed to pinworms (such as anal pruritus, anal skin lesions, enuresis, loss of appetite, masturbation, nausea and vomiting, vague intestinal pain, diarrhea, weight loss, vaginitis, and restlessness) was significantly more common in infected than in uninfected children [4]. Results were similar in a group of schoolchildren in South Dakota, and the general conclusion reached was that a large proportion of pinworm infections are essentially asymptomatic. It appears, however, that the symptoms of enterobiasis are related largely to perianal and perineal pruritus; these symptoms rapidly abate after treatment. The reasons why some individuals are symptomatic and most are not remain speculative but may be related to the intensity of infection, the psychiatric state of the infected individual and his family, or an allergic response to products of the parasite. In the last regard, it is interesting to note that of 90 individuals with pinworm, 37 showed an immediate dermal response

to adult and larval worm antigens of *E. vermicularis* [2].

Ectopic disease. There is evidence that *E. vermicularis* is not a tissue parasite. Thus neither the significant eosinophilia nor the raised level of serum reaginic antibody (IgE) usually noted in infections with tissue-invading helminths is found in enterobiasis. Nevertheless, case reports of ectopic tissue-invading pinworm adults, larvae, and eggs are continually appearing. In 1950 an exhaustive review of 103 citations on this subject was published [5], and more case reports have appeared since that time. When the vast numbers of infected individuals are considered, the number of cases reported has been miniscule. In general, one must agree with the conclusions reached in Symmer's review [5]: enterobiasis is occasionally associated with ulcerative lesions of the small and large intestines, but the association is probably coincidental; the infection is not a significant cause of appendicitis; only in exceptional cases do the worms cause pathologic changes in the tissues, and their

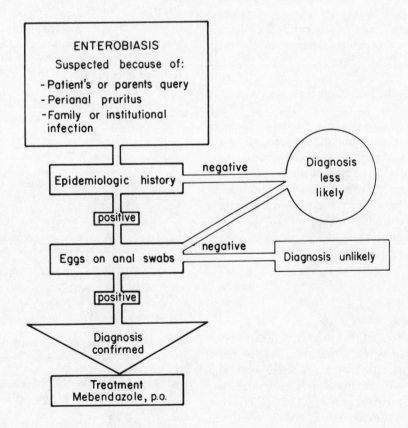

Figure 1. The progression to a definitive diagnosis of enterobiasis; p.o. = perorally.

pathogenicity in this respect is trivial; and the small numbers of cases in which *Enterobius*-containing nodules have been found in the female genitalia or peritoneum (the parasite having reached the peritoneal cavity through the genital tract) have rarely been associated with symptoms necessitating surgical intervention.

Diagnosis

The process involved in the diagnosis and management of enterobiasis is illustrated in the accompanying algorithm (figure 1). Pinworms can be seen with the naked eye, although they can easily be confused with bits of white thread. Thus, having spotted the putative worm, a patient or parent may either question the physician about it or bring in a specimen. Perianal pruritis in children with concomitant perineal irritation and restlessness or sleeplessness may suggest the diagnosis. Enterobiasis tends to run in families and is particularly common in institutions; an epidemiological history, therefore, is of value.

Pinworm eggs are relatively rarely seen in conventional stool examinations. They are more readily found by the following procedure. In the morning, immediately after the subject wakes up, the adhesive side of a 2-inch strip of cellophane tape is pressed repeatedly against the perianal skin. The tape is placed adhesive-side down onto a drop of toluene on a microscope slide, and the slide is scanned for adherent eggs at a magnification of ×100. The eggs are oval, flat on one side, and $50 \times 30~\mu m$ in size. A single test detects about 50% of infections, three tests detect 90%, and five tests detect 99%. When infection is detected in an individual, all members of the family should be examined.

Management

It should be reiterated that most individuals in our society have a strong fear of and aversion to parasitic worms. Therefore, after (or perhaps before) obtaining a positive diagnosis, the physician should immediately inform the patient of the prevalence of this infection, its complete lack of socioeconomic fastidiousness, and its harmlessness. Although it is frequently stated in textbooks that "personal cleanliness is essential" and a rigorous preventive schedule is usually recommended, this approach is probably useless [6] and tends to enhance the psychological trauma of the infection. Enterobiasis has not been controlled by the most stringently applied sanitary measures, including daily thorough cleansing of each room in the house, daily changing and sterilization of bedclothes and nightclothes, frequent brushing of nails, and two showers per day [6]. Furthermore, in spite of highly effective, single-dose anthelmintic therapy, reinfection occurs frequently. Thus in one study, when three doses of a drug were administered to families at spaced intervals to prevent reinfection, the prevalance of infection was only slightly reduced four months after treatment; the major source of reinfection appeared to be extrafamilial contacts [7]. It is recommended, therefore, that drug therapy be administered when pinworm infection is diagnosed and that treatment be reinstituted if and when symptoms return and eggs are again found in the perianal area.

A new oral, broad-spectrum antihelminthic drug, mebendazole (Vermox,® Ortho Pharmaceutical Corp., Raritan, N.J.) is recommended for treatment of enterobiasis. Absorption from the gastrointestinal tract is minimal, and no side effects have been reported [8]. A single oral dose of 100 mg (one pill) has resulted in cure rates of 90%–100%.

References

1. Warren, K. S. Helminthic diseases endemic in the United States. Am. J. Trop. Med. Hyg. 23:723–730, 1974.
2. Cram, E. B. Studies on oxyuriasis. XXVIII. Summary and conclusions. Am. J. Dis. Child. 65:46–59, 1943.
3. Mathies, A. W., Jr. *Enterobius vermicularis* infection. Certain aspects of the host-parasite relationship. Am. J. Dis. Child. 101:174–177, 1961.
4. Weller, T. H., Sorenson, C. W. Enterobiasis: its incidence and symptomatology in a group of 505 children. N. Engl. J. Med. 224:143–146, 1941.
5. Symmers, W. St. C. Pathology of oxyuriasis. Arch. Pathol. 50:475–516, 1950.
6. Sawitz, W., D'Antoni, J. S., Rhude, K., Lob, S. Studies on the epidemiology of oxyuriasis. South. Med. J. 33:913–921, 1940.
7. Matsen, J. M., Turner, J. A. Reinfection in enterobiasis (pinworm infection). Am. J. Dis. Child. 118:576–581, 1969.
8. Mebendazole—a new anthelmintic. Med. Lett. Drugs Ther. 17:37–38, 1975.

The Filariases

The filariases, a group of infections with round worms (nematodes) of the superfamily Filarioidea, constitute a major global health problem. Bancroftian filariasis is spread widely throughout the tropical world, as is the less common tropical pulmonary eosinophilia. Onchocerciasis is seen in Africa and in Central and South America. Malayan filariasis occurs only in southern and Southeast Asia, and loiasis is restricted to western Africa. None of these infections is endemic in the United States at present, but imported cases may be encountered.

The filariases are transmitted to man by the bite of infected insect vectors; mosquitoes transmit bancroftian and malayan filariasis, blackflies spread onchocerciasis, and tabanid flies are the vectors of loiasis. The injected larvae mature into adult worms that may be found (according to the species) in the lymphatic system, the connective tissues, the serous cavities, the chambers of the heart, or the pulmonary arteries. After mating, the adult worms release first-stage larvae (microfilariae) that may be found either in the tissues or in the blood.

The pathogenicity of the adults and the microfilariae varies according to the species of infecting worm. In bancroftian and malayan filariasis, the presence of adult worms in the lymph nodes and vessels is associated with inflammation and obstruction of the lymphatic system resulting in lymphadenitis, lymphedema, and elephantiasis, while the microfilariae, which circulate in the bloodstream, do not appear to be pathogenic. In contrast, microfilariae in the lungs may cause tropical pulmonary eosinophilia with cough, wheezing, and dyspnea. In onchocerciasis, the adult worms produce unsightly subcutaneous nodules, but the clinically important dermatitis and eye lesions are produced by the tissue-swelling microfilariae. In loiasis, skin swellings are thought to be associated with adult worms migrating through the connective tissues. In addition to the major filariases described above, there are a number of other human filarial parasites that are either of doubtful pathogenicity (e.g., *Dipetalonema perstans* and *Mansonella ozzardi*) or uncommon (e.g., *Dipetalonema streptocerca*). *Dirofilaria* species principally infect animals but have occasionally been found in man.

Definitive diagnosis requires the isolation and identification of the parasite, but it is often difficult to find either the adult worms or the microfilariae. Immunological diagnosis is unsatisfactory because serological tests and skin tests do not distinguish among the various filariases and because there is considerable cross-reactivity with other nematode infections. In some situations a drug-induced exacerbation or alleviation of signs and symptoms provides the only significant evidence of a filarial infection.

Treatment of the filariases is often unsatisfactory. The drug diethylcarbamazine destroys microfilariae, but its administration may be associated with severe allergic reactions. Moreover, this drug is of uncertain value in the therapy of bancroftian and malayan filariasis since microfilariae do not play a major role in the pathogenesis of these infections; neither is such therapy very effective in onchocerciasis or loiasis, in which adult worms survive to produce more larvae. Drugs such as suramin will destroy the adult worms of some species but may have severe toxic side effects. Finally, death of the worms may also bring about an exacerbation of symptoms.

Bancroftian and Malayan Filariasis

Bancroftian and malayan filariasis (often simply known as filariasis) results from mosquito-transmitted infection with the nematodes *Wuchereria bancrofti* or *Brugia malayi*. The larvae introduced by the insects mature into adults in the lymphatics; thus the clinical features are due to inflammation and obstruction of the lymphatic system. The fertilized females release large numbers of microfilariae, which circulate in the bloodstream for long periods or until they are ingested by a mosquito.

It is estimated that more than 250 million people are infected with these parasites. Bancroftian filariasis is spread widely throughout the tropical and subtropical regions of South America, Africa, southern and Southeast Asia, and the Pacific. Malayan filariasis is more restricted in distribution, being found only in southern and Southeast Asia. Bancroftian filariasis used to be endemic in the United States. In South

Carolina in 1915, microfilariae were found in 20% of 400 hospitalized patients, and one in four of these persons had a history suggestive of filarial disease. The last autochthonous case reported in the United States was in 1930. During World War II thousands of American troops serving in the Pacific were infected with *W. bancrofti* [1]. Fear of developing hydroceles and elephantiasis was intense, but chronic sequelae occurred in only a very small proportion of patients. Imported filariasis is occasionally seen in immigrants, especially from the Caribbean and Pacific Islands.

Life Cycle

Man is inoculated with the parasite when bitten by an infective mosquito. The larvae pass into the lymphatics and lymph nodes, where they develop to maturity during a period of six to twelve months. The white, thread-like adults of both sexes lie tightly intertwined in the lymphatics. The males of *W. bancrofti* are approximately 40 × 0.1 mm and the females 100 × 0.25 mm in size, whereas *B. malayi* are slightly smaller. The fertilized females discharge microfilariae, which pass via the lymphatics into the bloodstream; *W. bancrofti* microfilariae measure 260 × 8 μm, whereas those of *B. malayi* are 230 × 6 μm in size. In addition to size, there are also differences between the caudal nuclear pattern of the microfilariae of *W. bancroft* and those of *B. malayi*. When microfilariae are ingested in the mosquito's blood meal, they penetrate the thoracic muscles of the insect, where they undergo two moults and then migrate to the proboscis; the entire process takes from one to three weeks.

Epidemiology

In many patients with filariasis there is a surge of microfilariae into the peripheral blood around midnight. The mechanism of this phenomenon, which is known as nocturnal periodicity, is not completely understood. While most patients infected with *W. bancrofti* exhibit this periodicity, those infected in the South Pacific show a much less pronounced peak, which is maximal during the day. *B. malayi* infections show nocturnal peaks of various intensities.

Man is the only known host of *W. bancrofti*, but *B. malayi* has also been found in primates and felines. A large number of rural and urban species of mosquito have been shown to transmit the parasite. The biting times of the mosquitoes usually coincide with the periodic microfilaremia of the parasite. Transmission in a given area depends upon the presence of suitable vectors in large enough numbers and an adequate reservoir of circulating microfilariae. In a study in Rangoon, Burma, each person was exposed to approximately 80,000 bites per year of which 300 (0.4%) were by infective mosquitoes. It was calculated that an average of 15,500 bites from infective mosquitoes were necessary to produce one case of microfilaremia [2]. A study undertaken in Calcutta, India showed a similar total number of bites per year but approximately four times as many infective bites and four times as high an incidence of microfilaremia [3]. It seems likely that patent infections are produced only when a susceptible individual receives a large number of infective larvae and that obstructive disease develops only when exposure continues for many years.

Disease Syndromes

Many patients in endemic areas have asymptomatic infections. A study in Calcutta showed that only 0.7% of the adult male population had severe lymphedema and 2.2% had large hydroceles, despite a microfilaremia rate of 20–25% [3]. Similarly, a survey of 178 Samoan immigrants to the United States showed that 14% had microfilaremia, but only a small proportion had clinical features of filariasis. Conversely, clinical disease may be found in the absence of microfilaremia. Thousands of American army and navy personnel stationed in the South Pacific during World War II developed early filariasis with epididymitis, orchitis, lymphangitis, and lymphadenitis; microfilariae were rarely present in the blood, although worms were found in specimens from 22% of 364 reported biopsies [1]. Furthermore, microfilariae are not usually found in the blood of patients with advanced filariasis.

(1) Acute inflammatory reactions. In bancroftian filariasis, patients may present with an acute lymphangitis or lymphadenitis, usually of the lower limbs. Funiculitis, epididymitis, and orchitis are also common and may be associated with the rapid develop-

ment of a hydrocele. In malayan filariasis, the upper limbs are more frequently affected, and involvement of the genitalia is less common. Headache, backache, and nausea are often symptoms in both forms, and fever may occur. The acute episodes usually subside after a few days to a few weeks but frequently recur. Persistent generalized lymphadenopathy is often seen.

(2) Chronic obstructive lesions. Continued residence in an endemic area, with recurrent inflammatory episodes and subsequent fibrosis, may lead to the development of lymphatic obstruction. If enough vessels are involved, lymphedema will develop, and lymphatic varices may arise, especially in the femoral, inguinal, and testicular regions. The skin and subcutaneous tissues of the scrotum may become swollen, and effusion of fluid in the tunica vaginalis may lead to a chronic hydrocele. Obstruction of deeply sited lymphatics may result in chylous ascites and in pleural or joint effusions. Chyluria develops when swollen lymphatics burst into the urinary tract. Persistent edema of skin and hypodermis leads to elephantiasis characterized by thickening of the subcutaneous tissue, hypertrophy of the epithelium, development of warty excrescences, irregular foldings, and secondary infections.

Diagnosis

An algorithm illustrating the sequence of steps necessary for the diagnosis of filariasis is presented in figure 1. The presence of microfilariae in the blood does not necessarily denote filarial disease but may simply indicate an asymptomatic carrier. The algorithm is constructed from the point of view of patients with either acute symptomatology (such as lymphangitis, lymphadenopathy, funiculitis, and epididymitis) or signs of chronic lymphatic obstruction (such as hydrocele, chyluria, or elephantiasis). In either case, a geographic history must be taken. If the patient has never been to or has resided only transiently in an endemic area, the diagnosis is unlikely. If the geographic history is positive, microfilariae should be sought in the blood although they are rarely found in either the early or the advanced stages of the disease.

A blood sample taken at midnight will detect all forms of the parasites, whether or not there is nocturnal periodicity. A concentration technique is most effective. Blood (1 ml) is diluted in 10 ml of 4% formalin in water, shaken for hemolysis of the red cells, and centrifuged for 5 min at 1,000 rpm (400 g). The deposit is spread on a glass slide, dried, fixed in methanol for 3 min, dried again, and stained for 30 min with 10% Giemsa in phosphate buffer (Giemsa stain, Fisher Scientific, Fairlawn, N.J.). New, highly sensitive techniques have been developed for the detection of microfilariae, but these methods are of most value for epidemiological studies. For routine diagnosis of individual infection in hospital laboratories, the established techniques are simpler, allow species identification, and provide a permanent record. Microfilariae may occasionally be seen in chylous urine or hydrocele fluid.

Although the differentiation of *W. bancrofti* from *B. malayi* is not critical to the diagnosis, these two types of microfilariae must be distinguished from those of other filariae whose larvae circulate in the blood. The microfilariae of *Loa loa* are also found in the peripheral blood. *D. perstans* is widely distributed throughout Africa and South America, and *M. ozzardi* is found in South America. The adult worms are found in the serous cavities and produce microfilaremia; the larvae are transmitted by biting midges (*Culicoides*). The vast majority of infections are asymptomatic, although eosinophilia is common. Treatment is unnecessary. Microfilariae are distinguished on the basis of the presence or absence of a sheath, the shape of the tail, and the pattern of nuclei within the tail. A key for species identification is available [4]. Failure to find microfilariae may necessitate lymph node or vessel biopsy, but adult worms are found in only about 25% of specimens.

In the absence of a parasitological diagnosis, serological tests may be considered. These tests are performed by the Mycology and Parasitology Section, Center for Disease Control, Atlanta, Ga. Immunological tests for filariasis, however, are not highly specific in that they do not differentiate among the various filariases and other nematode infections. Eosinophilia is not a reliable indicator of infection and is of little help in making the diagnosis. If the filariae cannot be identified, the diagnosis must be made on clinical grounds by the exclusion of other causes.

Management

Treatment with diethylcarbamazine citrate (Hetra-

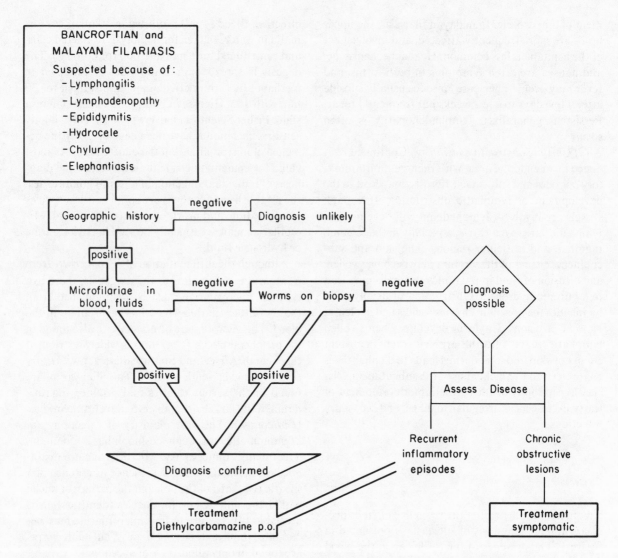

Figure 1. The progression to a diagnosis of bancroftian and malayan filariasis; p.o. = perorally.

zan,® Lederle, Pearl River, N.Y.) rapidly reduces the number of microfilariae in the peripheral blood. This response may be permanent, a fact suggesting that the drug may kill or sterilize the adult worms. Further episodes of lymphangitis are sometimes prevented, but established elephantiasis or hydrocele will not regress. The drug is given initially in small doses because of reactions to dying microfilariae, as manifested by fever, malaise, headache, backache, nausea, and vomiting. After several days of treatment, some patients develop an inflammatory reaction in a lymph node or vessel, presumably around a dead or dying worm. Diethylcarbamazine is administered orally after meals in a three-week course as follows: day 1, 50 mg; day 2, 50 mg three times; day 3, 100 mg three times; days 4–21, 3 mg/kg three times daily. Treat-

ment of symptoms includes rest and administration of anti-inflammatory and analgesic drugs. Mild lymphedema may be controlled with elastic stockings. Advanced hydrocele requires surgery.

Patients with early filariasis or asymptomatic microfilaremia should be strongly reassured that the likelihood of developing long-term sequelae is remote. Patients who are returning to an endemic area should institute measures of vector control such as screens, mosquito nets, and insect repellents.

Tropical Pulmonary Eosinophilia

Tropical pulmonary eosinophilia (TPE, tropical eosinophilia with eosinophilic lung) is a syndrome that consists of a chronic paroxysmal cough, eosinophilia, abnormal chest X ray, and a positive therapeutic response to treatment with diethylcarbamazine. TPE is due to microfilariae of uncertain origin in the tissues, especially in the lungs, but diagnosis is difficult since there are no circulating microfilariae. TPE has a distribution similar to that of bancroftian and malayan filariasis and is most commonly seen in southern Asia; it has also been recorded in Africa and South America.

Life Cycle

The worms responsible for TPE have not been definitely identified, and thus the complete life cycle of the organism is unknown. Microfilariae have been found in the lungs, lymph nodes, and liver [5], but the adult worms have so far remained elusive. It is uncertain whether the illness represents an unusual reaction to larvae of *Wuchereria* or *Brugia* species or a reaction to a worm such as *Dirofilaria,* which is usually a parasite of animals.

Epidemiology

TPE has most frequently been described in areas endemic for bancroftian and malayan filariases. TPE also is presumably transmitted by mosquitoes. Nevertheless, patients with pulmonary infiltrates and eosinophilia are found in the United States, where *Dirofilaria* infections of dogs are common. It is possible, therefore, that the condition occurs in the United States but has hitherto been unrecognized.

Disease Syndromes

The onset is usually insidious, with a dry cough that becomes paroxysmal and worse at night. The cough may become productive, and some patients have small hemoptyses. Wheezing and dyspnea may occur. Frequently, there are nonspecific features such as malaise, fatigue, anorexia, and weight loss, Physical examination may yield negative results but often reveals scattered rhonchi and crepitations. Some patients have mild hepatomegaly or lymphadenopathy. These features usually persist for many months, although severity may fluctuate. A variant of the syndrome occurs in which there is persistent eosinophilia with unidentified microfilariae in the lymph nodes

and spleen, but microfilariae are again absent from the blood.

Diagnosis

An algorithm for diagnosis and management of TPE is outlined in figure 2. The patient may present because of pulmonary symptoms or eosinophilia. If the patient has not been to an endemic area, the diagnosis is unlikely. Eosinophilia occurs in all cases, usually with > 2,000 cells/μl. Chest X ray is abnormal in 98% of patients [6]. Translucency of the mid-zonal lung fields is reduced, often with reticulonodular opacities or hilar prominence with perihilar striation and a peripheral net-like pattern. Serological tests for filariasis are performed by the Center for Disease Control, Atlanta, Ga. Although nonspecific, the tests usually yield positive results for TPE. In many cases the final arbiter is a therapeutic trial with diethylcarbamazine; failure of response renders the diagnosis unlikely. Although many patients have been diagnosed by a lung biopsy that shows an eosinophilic granulomatous reaction with or without microfilariae, a presumptive clinical diagnosis can be made and then established by a satisfactory response to diethylcarbamazine.

Pulmonary infiltrates with eosinophilia occur in several other helminthic infections. *Ascaris lumbricoides, Strongyloides stercoralis,* and hookworm larvae may produce such a picture as they migrate through the lungs. In these infections symptoms usually last for only a few days; in contrast, TPE tends to be a chronic, recurrent disease.

Management

Administration of diethylcarbamazine orally in a dose of 3 mg/kg three times daily for two weeks is an effective form of treatment. There may be fever and exacerbation of symptoms during the first few days of therapy. The eosinophil level falls and the chest X ray clears over a few weeks. Relapses may occur but usually respond to a second course of therapy.

Onchocerciasis

Onchocerciasis is caused by the filarial worm *Onchocerca volvulus,* which is transmitted by simuliid

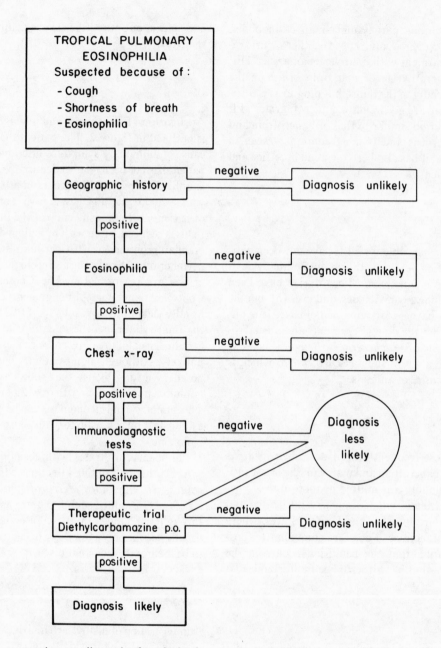

Figure 2. The progression to a diagnosis of tropical pulmonary eosinophilia; p.o. = perorally.

blackflies. In contrast to most other filariases, both adult worms and microfilariae are found in the tissues rather than in the blood. The presence of adults is manifested by cutaneous nodules, and the microfilariae by an itchy dermatitis and eye lesions that may eventuate in blindness [7].

In Africa, 30 million people living in rain forest and savannah regions stretching from Senegal to Ethiopia in the north and from Angola to Tanzania in the south

are infected by *O. volvulus*. The infection is also found in Central and South America; nearly one million people are affected in Guatemala, Venezuela, and Colombia. There are some epidemiological and clinical differences between the infections on the two continents. Onchocerciasis is sometimes seen in the United States either in visitors and migrants from endemic areas or in Americans who have resided in such areas.

Life Cycle

Man is infected by the bite of female blackflies of the genus *Simulium*. The larvae penetrate the skin and migrate into the connective tissues, where they develop into white, filiform adult worms during a period of 12 months. The males (20–40 × 0.2 mm) and females (350–500 × 0.3 mm) are found together in nodules of fibrous tissue, where they may live as long as 15 years. Each female produces large numbers of microfilariae, which are unsheathed and measure 140–350 × 5–9 μm. They migrate through the tissues where they may live for up to two years. After ingestion by a fly, the larvae pass to the thoracic muscles where two moults occur; by the 10th day the infective third-stage larvae are found at the base of the labrum.

Epidemiology

Man is the only known definitive host of *O. volvulus*. Onchocerciasis tends to be focal in distribution within its endemic areas. The pattern of infection is determined by variations in the parasite, vectors, and host response. The strains of *O. volvulus* in America differ from those in Africa, and there is also variation (according to area) within Africa. Moreover, the breeding and biting habits of the vectors considerably influence the prevalence and pattern of disease.

In Africa the flies breed in fast-running streams and rivers and tend to bite low on the body. In the rain forest transmission occurs throughout the year and is associated with gross skin lesions, but in the savannah transmission may be seasonal, and eye lesions are more prevalent.

In America the flies breed in small, even minute, streams. The main vector in Guatemala tends to bite on the upper parts of the body; this fact may explain the greater frequency of head nodules and eye lesions in this area.

Disease Syndromes

Many of the indigenous inhabitants of regions with a low or moderate prevalence of *O. volvulus* have asymptomatic infections. In areas of high prevalence and intensity of infection, signs and symptoms of disease may be common [8]. Expatriates who contract onchocerciasis often suffer greatly from pruritis, even though the worm burden may be light and microfilariae are difficult to find.

(1) Nodules. Firm, nontender fibrous nodules with freely moving overlying skin may be found; these nodules vary in size from several millimeters to several centimeters. The number of nodules varies greatly, as does their distribution over the body. In the African form of the disease, the majority of nodules are located over the bony prominences, especially the pelvis, lateral chest wall, spine, and knees. In Central America they tend to occur on the upper part of the body, especially the head.

(2) Dermatitis. Involvement of the skin often begins with intense itching, and scratching may lead to secondary infection. A papular rash is frequently seen on the buttocks. Mottled depigmentation may occur. More severe disease is characterized by cutaneous lymphedema (especially of the trunk), which may be followed by a leathery thickening of the skin. Finally, atrophy with loss of elasticity gives a prematurely aged appearance. Lymphadenopathy is common, and patients in Africa are prone to develop "hanging groin," pendulous sacs containing inguinal and femoral lymph nodes.

Patients in Central America may develop erythematous lesions of the face or upper trunk, a purplish eruption on the upper part of the body resembling lichen planus, or a leonine facies.

(3) Eye lesions. Impaired visual acuity or blindness is the most serious complication of onchocerciasis and usually takes many years to develop. Microfilariae can often be seen in the anterior chamber or cornea with a slit lamp and may be the only sign of eye involvement. The earliest and by far the most common lesions are punctate keratitis or snowflake opacities of the cornea, which may be followed by pannus formation and corneal fibrosis. Atrophy of the iris is common, and occasionally an acute iridocyclitis is seen. Posterior synechiae may develop and may be followed by secondary glaucoma or cataract. Choroidoretinitis, which may be extensive, has been reported in some patients, and optic atrophy may be found.

Diagnosis

The diagnosis and management of onchocerciasis is

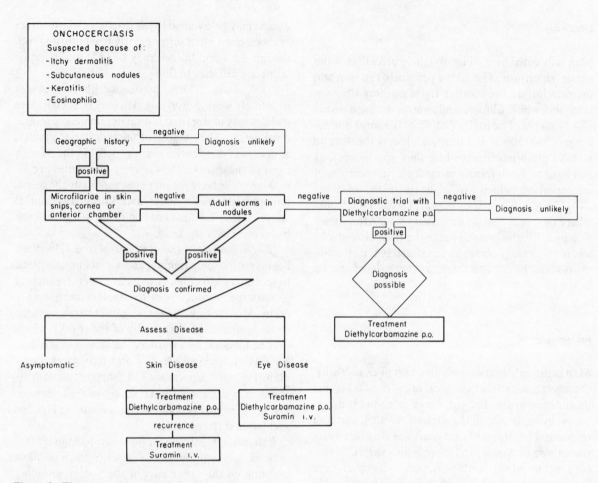

Figure 3. The progression to a diagnosis of onchocerciasis; p.o. = perorally; i.v. = intravenously.

illustrated in the accompanying algorithm (figure 3). The infection may be suspected in a patient who presents with itchy dermatitis or subcutaneous nodules or with eye lesions such as keratitis, iritis, or choroiditis. Onchocerciasis may also be considered in the differential diagnosis of eosinophilia. If the patient has not been in an endemic area, the diagnosis is essentially ruled out. If the geographic history is positive, however, a search should be made for microfilariae in skin snips and in the anterior chamber and cornea by means of a slit lamp.

Skin snips are taken by raising small cones of skin about 3 mm in diameter with the tip of a needle, then cutting them off with a razor blade. They should be taken from the thighs, buttocks, and over the iliac crests and scapulae. The snips are placed in drops of 0.9% NaCl, teased and allowed to stand for half an hour, and then examined under a microscope for microfilariae. The snip should be bloodless; otherwise there may be confusion with microfilariae of *L. loa*

or *D. perstans* [4]. Microfilariae found in the skin of patients from tropical rain forest areas of western Africa must be differentiated from those of *D. streptocerca,* which may also cause dermatitis [9]. Microfilariae may also be found in the urine of up to 30% of patients on both continents. Sometimes fluid can be aspirated from a nodule and microfilariae found on microscopy. The diagnosis may also be made by excision of a nodule and identification of the adult worms by histological examination.

Eosinophilia is common and may reach very high levels. Immunological tests are of no help in making the diagnosis since they do not differentiate among the various filariases and cross-react with other nematode infections.

If nodules are not present and no microfilariae are found, the response to a single oral 50-mg dose of diethylcarbamazine can be assessed (Mazzotti test). If an acute exacerbation of the rash occurs 1–24 hr later or a rash appears in a patient who was previously without skin symptoms, the diagnosis is likely but unproven. If this and all other tests yield negative results, the diagnosis is unlikely.

Management

(1) Chemotherapy. The treatment of onchocerciasis is unsatisfactory since the available drugs can be toxic. The two drugs most commonly used are diethylcarbamazine, which kills the microfilariae but has little effect on the adult worms, and suramin, which kills the adult worms and some of the microfilariae [10].

It is probably wise to treat all symptomatic expatriates, but the recommended regimen varies according to whether the diagnosis has been parasitologically proven, whether the eyes are involved, and whether there are any contraindications to treatment with suramin.

(a) Asymptomatic infection. Patients with proven onchocerciasis who are asymptomatic need not be treated, but it is wise to review the patient periodically for several years, particularly with reference to the development of eye lesions.

(b) Skin disease. Patients with skin disease only should be treated with diethylcarbamazine. If the symptoms continue to recur after several courses of diethylcarbamazine and the diagnosis has been parasitologically proven, suramin should be administered. Patients who have a positive Mazzotti test but in whom parasites have never been found should be treated only with diethylcarbamazine.

(c) Eye disease. Patients with eye disease should be treated with diethylcarbamazine followed by suramin. In patients with renal disease, diethylcarbamazine alone is given, but repeated courses may be necessary.

In view of the severe reactions that may occur with diethylcarbamazine (such as fever, rash, generalized body pains, conjunctivitis, and iritis), the dose is built up gradually as described in the section on bancroftian filariasis. In the case of suramin (Antrypol, Moranyl, Parasitic Drug Service of the Center for Disease Control, Atlanta, Ga.), a test dose of 100 mg is given initially for detection of the rare patient with an idiosyncratic reaction such as vomiting and collapse. One gram is then given iv each week for six weeks. If proteinuria at a level of >20 mg/100 ml or abundant casts appear in the urine, the drug should be stopped. An exfoliative dermatitis sometimes develops for which corticosteroid therapy may be necessary.

(2) Nodulectomy. Where practicable, it may be worthwhile to remove all identifiable nodules, particularly in patients with the American form of the disease, since such removal reduces the chances of eye lesions.

(3) Ophthalmic treatment. In addition to antiparasitic therapy, expert ophthalmological advice should be sought for the management of patients with onchocercal eye disease.

Loiasis

Loiasis is an infection with the filarial worm *Loa loa,* which is transmitted by biting tabanid flies. The adult parasites reside in the subcutaneous connective tissues; the major clinical manifestations are transient, so-called calabar swellings. Occasionally, the adult worm migrates through the subconjunctival tissues, where it may be directly visualized. The microfilariae that circulate in the blood have not been associated with any specific signs or symptoms.

Loiasis is irregularly distributed in western and central Africa from the Gulf of Guinea to Lakes Victoria and Tanganyika; the disease is most prevalent in eastern Nigeria, the Cameroon Republic, and Zaire. Imported cases have been reported in the United States.

Life Cycle

Man is infected by the bite of female tabanid flies of the genus *Chrysops.* The larvae penetrate the skin and migrate into the connective tissues, where they develop during the next 12 months into white, thread-like, cylindrical worms (30–70 × 0.3 mm). After maturation and reproduction, the larvae, surrounded by a sheath and measuring 300 × 8 μm, are found in the blood during the day. After ingestion by the fly, the microfilariae pass into the thoracic muscles, where they undergo three moults; after two weeks they make their way to the base of the proboscis, ready for transmission.

Epidemiology

Man is probably the only definitive host of *L. loa.* The

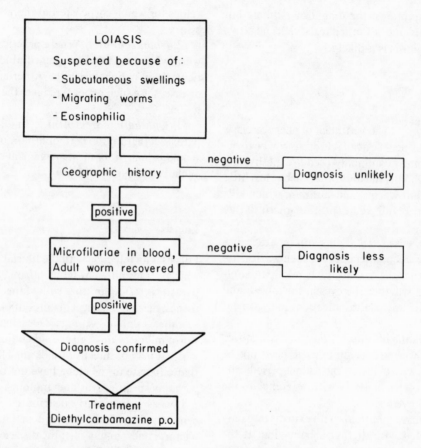

Figure 4.   The progression to a diagnosis of loiasis; p.o. = perorally.

vectors are day-biting flies that live in the canopy of
the rain forest and lay their eggs in the wet mud
swamps and river edges below the forest trees. The
infection is therefore much more prevalent among the
inhabitants of the rain forest than among those of the
savannah. The flies have specific biting habits, in that
they are attracted by dark skin and clothing, wood-
smoke, and movements and do most of their biting in
the shade at the edges of the open spaces of the rain
forest.

Disease Syndromes

Many subjects with loiasis are asymptomatic. Eosinophilia is common and may reach very high levels.
Patients with overt clinical manifestations usually
present in one of two ways, the first being far more
common.

(1) Calabar swellings.   These transient swellings
are areas of localized subcutaneous edema. They may
occur anywhere but are especially common around
medium-sized joints and in areas exposed to trauma,
such as the legs, hands, and orbits. The onset of the
lesions is often heralded by local pain or itching for
1–2 hr; an edematous, nonerythematous swelling
10–20 cm in diameter then develops, lasts for several
days, and slowly subsides. These swellings recur irregularly either at the same site or in various locations.

(2) Worm migration.   The adult worms occasionally migrate under the skin producing a prickly,
crawling sensation. When they pass under the ocular
or palpebral conjunctiva, where they may be directly
visualized, they produce an intense, edematous conjunctivitis that may last for several days.

Diagnosis

The diagnosis and management of loiasis is illustrated
in the accompanying algorithm (figure 4). The in-

fection should be suspected in a patient who presents with recurrent, localized edematous skin lesions or with a history of prickly, creeping sensations in the skin. Occasionally, the worm may have been seen in the subconjunctiva. Loiasis should also be considered in the differential diagnosis of eosinophilia, which may reach high levels in this helminthic infection. The diagnosis is virtually ruled out if the patient has not been to rural areas of western or central Africa. If the geographic history is positive, a search should be made for microfilariae in a specimen of blood by the method described in the section on bancroftian filariasis. In this case, however, best results are achieved when the sample is taken during the daytime (10 A.M.–2 P.M.). Failure to find microfilariae does not rule out the diagnosis. If the adult worm is seen, an attempt should be made to excise it. Immunological tests are not helpful, since *L. loa* cross-reacts with other nematodes as well as with other filarial worms.

Treatment

Although diethylcarbamazine may eliminate microfilariae from the blood, its effect on the adult worms is less certain. The drug is administered orally as described in the section on bancroftian filariasis and is given in small doses because of reactions to dying microfilariae, including fever, malaise, swelling of joints, and headache. In the event of a severe reaction to therapy, the drug should be stopped and corticosteroids given if necessary. Symptoms may recur and require additional courses of treatment with diethylcarbamazine.

Dirofilariasis

Dirofilariasis is a zoonotic infection. Several *Dirofilaria* species that infect animals may occasionally be found in man; the two most common are *Dirofilaria immitis* and *Dirofilaria tenuis* (*Dirofilaria conjunctivae*). Most cases have been reported from the United States, particularly from Florida, but others have been described in Europe, Asia, Africa, and Oceania.

Life Cycle

The adult worms of *D. immitis* are normally found in the right heart and pulmonary arteries of dogs and may be up to 25 cm in length and several millimeters in diameter. Unsheathed microfilariae (320 μm long) are released by fertilized females and pass into the bloodstream, where they may be ingested by various species of mosquito. After incubation for two weeks, third-stage larvae are found at the base of the proboscis, ready for transmission. Man is a poor host, and in the rare case in which adult worms develop, microfilariae are not found in the bloodstream.

Epidemiology

It is increasingly evident that *D. immitis* is spread widely throughout many of the temperate and tropical countries of the world and that human infection may occur wherever man, mosquitoes, and infected dogs are closely associated. Canine dirofilariasis is spread throughout much of the eastern half of the United States and in scattered areas of the rest of North America. *D. tenuis* has been found in raccoons.

Disease Syndromes, Diagnosis, and Management

There are two common clinical presentations, both of which may be associated with eosinophilia [11].

(1) Pulmonary lesions. Pulmonary lesions are usually produced by *D. immitis,* the heartworm of dogs. In man, the worm is usually seen in the heart or the lungs. It may be found incidentally at postmortem examination. Clinical manifestations of *D. immitis* infection of the lungs may include cough or chest pain or a solitary coin-type lesion that is noted on chest X ray. Diagnosis and treatment may occur simultaneously by surgical excision of the lesion.

(2) Subcutaneous lesions. Subcutaneous lesions are usually produced by *D. tenuis.* Most patients present with a subcutaneous nodule that may have been present for several weeks before becoming inflamed. The nodules may be found anywhere, are occasionally migratory, and usually do not recur. Diagnosis and treatment are by excision.

References

1. Wartman, W. B. Filariasis in American armed forces in World War II. Medicine (Balt.) 26:333–394, 1947.

2. Hairston, N. G., De Meillon, B. On the inefficiency of trans-
    mission of *Wuchereria bancrofti* from mosquito to human
    host. Bull. W.H.O. 38:935–941, 1968.

3. Gubler, D. J., Bhattacharya, N. C. A quantitative approach
    to the study of Bancroftian filariasis. Am. J. Trop. Med.
    Hyg. 23:1027–1036, 1974.

4. Harder, H. I., Watson, D. Human filariasis: identification of
    species on the basis of staining and other morphologic
    characteristics of microfilariae. Am. J. Clin. Pathol. 42:
    333–339, 1964.

5. Webb, J. K. G., Job, C. K., Gault, E. W. Tropical eosinophilia:
    demonstration of microfilariae in lung, liver, and lymph
    nodes. Lancet 1:835–842, 1960.

6. Herlinger, H. Pulmonary changes in tropical eosinophilia. Br.
    J. Radiol. 36:889–901, 1963.

7. Nelson, G. S. Onchocerciasis. Adv. Parasitol. 8:173–224,
    1970.

8. Anderson, J., Fuglsang, H., Hamilton, P. J. S., Marshall, T.
    F. de C. Studies on onchocerciasis in the United Cameroon
    Republic. I. Comparison of populations with and without
    Onchocerca volvulus. Trans. R. Soc. Trop. Med. Hyg.
    68:190–208, 1974.

9. Meyers, W. M., Connor, D. H., Harman, L. E., Fleshman, K.,
    Moris, R., Neafie, R. C. Human streptocerciasis: a clin-
    ico-pathologic study of 40 Africans (Zairians) including
    identification of the adult filaria. Am. J. Trop. Med. Hyg.
    21:528–545, 1972.

10. Duke, B. O. L. The effects of drugs on *Onchocerca volvulus*.
    3. Trials of suramin at different dosages and a comparison
    of the brands Antrypol, Moranyl and Neganol. Bull.
    W.H.O. 39:157–167, 1968.

11. Beaver, P. C., Orihel, T. C. Human infection with filariae
    of animals in the United States. Am. J. Trop. Med. Hyg.
    14:1010–1029, 1965.

Liver, Intestinal, and Lung Flukes

Trematodes or flukes are parasitic flatworms with a unique life cycle involving sexual reproduction in the human definitive host and asexual reproduction in the intermediate host, the snail. These organisms are characterized by their final habitats in the definitive host according to the following four anatomic categories: *(1)* the bisexual blood flukes (*Schistosoma*), which live in the intestinal or vesical venules and infect man by direct penetration through the skin (see pp. 106–111); *(2)* the hermaphroditic liver flukes, which reside in the bile ducts and infect man by ingestion of watercress (*Fasciola*) or raw fish (*Clonorchis* and *Opisthorchis*); *(3)* the hermaphroditic intestinal fluke (*Fasciolopsis*), which infects man by ingestion of water chestnuts; and *(4)* the hermaphroditic lung fluke (*Paragonimus*), which infects man by ingestion of raw crabs or crayfish. The hermaphroditic trematodes have unique geographic distributions related either to the presence of the snail intermediate hosts or the dietary habits of the human definitive host.

Fascioliasis is a cosmopolitan zoonosis, and sporadic cases in humans appear in most areas of the world. The remainder of the hermaphroditic fluke infections of man are confined largely to Asia. It is important to note that the flukes do not multiply in man, that the intensity of infection is related to the degree of exposure to the infective larvae, that in most endemic areas the majority of cases have light or moderate worm burdens, and that overt disease occurs largely in the relatively small proportion of those with heavy worm burdens. It is unlikely that the average traveler would have a major and prolonged exposure to the infective larvae of these parasites, although immigrants from Asia may be heavily infected and have clinically overt disease.

Life Cycle

The flukes are called digenetic trematodes because they undergo two different modes of reproduction: sexual in the definitive host (man) and asexual in the intermediate host (snails). This exceedingly complex life cycle was first worked out for *Fasciola hepatica,* a liver fluke, which predominantly infects ruminants such as cattle and sheep and incidentally infects man. This inch-long hermaphroditic flatworm (30 × 13 mm) resides in the bile ducts of the liver where it produces 20,000 eggs per day for a period of many years. The large, yellow, operculated (having a lid) eggs (150 × 80 μm) pass into the lumen of the small intestine and out of the body in the feces. On entering freshwater, the eggs undergo a period of maturation and then hatch into ciliated miracidia. When these organisms find and penetrate certain species of snails, the miracidia undergo several developmental stages, multiplying eventually into large numbers of cercariae. These tailed, free-swimming organisms leave the snail and encyst as metacercariae on the leaves of freshwater plants. When ingested by the definitive host, the larvae excyst within a period of 48 hr, penetrate through the gut wall into the peritoneal cavity, and enter the liver through its capsule. The young flukes, 0.3 mm in length, then begin to wander through the tissues of the liver. This migratory phase continues for about six to nine weeks, after which the half-grown flukes penetrate the bile ducts where they mature and begin to produce eggs.

Clonorchis sinensis, Opisthorchis felineus, and *Opisthorchis viverrini* are also liver flukes, and, although their life cycle is similar to that of *Fasciola,* there are some very important differences. The relatively small, yellow operculated eggs (30 × 14 μm) are fully embryonated when they pass out of the body. The eggs hatch only after ingestion by certain species of snails, within which they develop into large numbers of motile, free-swimming cercariae. On coming into contact with certain freshwater fish, the cercariae penetrate under the scales or into the flesh, where they encyst as metacercariae. After ingestion of raw or inadequately cooked fish by a variety of mammalian hosts, the organisms excyst within the duodenum, and, in contrast to *F. hepatica,* the larvae pass directly into the bile ducts through the ampulla of Vater, where *Clonorchis* mature into 20 × 5-mm adult worms; *Opisthorchis* are somewhat smaller.

The life cycle of *Fasciolopsis buski,* the intestinal fluke, shares the same characteristics as *F. hepatica* in that the operculated eggs (130 × 80 μm) produced at a rate of about 25,000 per worm per day pass out of the body in an unembryonated state, the miracidia penetrate snails, and the cercariae encyst on certain species of water plants. The metacercariae excyst within the duodenum, become attached to the nearby intestinal wall, and develop into adult worms (50 × 40 mm) in about three months.

The golden brown, operculated eggs (100 × 60 μm) of *Paragonimus westermani,* the lung fluke, pass into the bronchioles, are coughed up, and are either voided in the sputum or swallowed and passed in the feces. These eggs also require a period of embryonation in the external environment; the miracidia then hatch and penetrate into suitable species of snails. The cercariae subsequently shed by the snails attack various species of freshwater crayfish and crabs and encyst as metacercariae in the tissues. After ingestion by the definitive host of raw or pickled crustacea or uncooked sauces made from them, the metacercariae excyst in the duodenum, penetrate the intestinal wall, and enter the peritoneal cavity from whence they migrate through the diaphragm and pleural cavity into the lungs. After a period of from several days to several weeks, the flukes finally lodge in the vicinity of the bronchioles where they develop into adult worms (10 × 5 mm) within tissue capsules laid down by the host. The circuitous route of migration through the host tissues may lead to the development of worms in ectopic sites, the most important being the brain.

Epidemiology

F. hepatica infection occurs worldwide in ruminants and has been associated with significant morbidity and mortality in domesticated animals such as sheep and cattle. For the most part, infection of man is sporadic and only a few hundred cases have been reported in the world's literature, usually in association with ingestion of wild watercress [1, 2]. Infection with *F. hepatica* is enzootic in most areas of the United States, although infection of humans seems to be exceedingly rare. Fascioliasis in man has almost always been identified during the acute migratory stage of infection; occasionally, worms are found in the bile ducts at surgery or autopsy. Recently, foci of chronic human fascioliasis have been found in the rural areas of Peru [3].

C. sinensis, O. felineus, and *O. viverrini* are common liver flukes of cats and dogs but also infect many other mammalian hosts. Although man is essentially an incidental host, millions of individuals are infected with these organisms. Clonorchiasis is prevalent in

China, Hong Kong, Vietnam, Korea, and Taiwan. Infection of humans with *O. felineus* has been reported in many parts of Southeast Asia and Asia as well as Eastern Europe and the U.S.S.R., and *O. viverrini* is prevalent in Thailand. Infection occurs after ingestion of raw or inadequately cooked or pickled freshwater fish (saltwater fish do not carry these parasites).

F. buski is a common parasite of man and pigs in the Far East and Southeast Asia. Infection in man is due to the consumption of raw pods, roots, stems, or bulbs of certain water plants and is related to peeling of the metacercaria-infested hull of these vegetables with the teeth prior to consumption.

Although *P. westermani* has a cosmopolitan distribution among mammals, infection in man is chiefly confined to the Far East but has been reported in Africa and South and Central America. Dietary habits are a major factor in the distribution of this infection in man, because paragonimiasis is transmitted by eating raw freshwater crayfish or crabs. Pickling these crustaceans in brine or crushing them for use as a sauce does not prevent infection. Recently, a relatively large number of cases has been reported in Nigeria; these cases were associated with the famine that occurred during the civil war several years ago.

Within man, the trematodes do not undergo direct replication but produce large numbers of eggs which pass out of the body in the feces, urine, or sputum. Thus, humans have different intensities of infection related largely to exposure to the infected larvae, i.e., frequency of consumption of contaminated foods. Mathematical models suggest that the intensity of infection in mammalian populations follows a negative binomial distribution and that the largest proportion of individuals have light to moderate infections. In recent years, controlled studies have been performed and have revealed that most infected individuals show no overt signs or symptoms of disease. Significant disease, whether hepatic, intestinal, or pulmonary, occurs largely in the small proportion of individuals who are infected with large numbers of flukes.

Disease Syndromes

Fascioliasis in man and animals has two distinct clinical phases. The first occurs in the initial six to nine weeks of infection when the larvae are migrating within the liver, and the second period begins when the larvae enter the bile ducts. The acute clinical syndrome is characterized by prolonged fever, pain in the right hypochondrium, and, sometimes, hepatomegaly, asthenia, and urticaria; a marked eosinophilia is usually seen during this period [1]. Asymptomatic acute infection has been reported in England [2] and seems to be common in Peru [3]. After the flukes enter the bile ducts, the symptoms appear to decline and disappear completely. Although animals with particularly heavy worm burdens may develop chronic biliary tract disease, this condition has been extremely rarely reported in man and even then is almost invariably an incidental finding at surgery or autopsy.

In contrast to fascioliasis, clonorchiasis and opisthorchiasis are not manifested by an acute syndrome, as the larval flukes do not undergo a migratory phase in the liver but enter directly into the bile ducts through the ampulla of Vater. The vast majority of individuals with infections due to *Clonorchis* and *Opisthorchis* show no significant signs or symptoms of disease when compared with uninfected matched control groups [4–6]. Pathological studies have revealed no gross changes in the liver in milder early infections. Despite the generally negative findings obtained in field populations, in highly endemic areas patients with chronic disease may filter through to hospital centers. These individuals suffer largely from cholangitis, cholangiohepatitis, and cholangiocarcinoma [7, 8].

Fasciolopsiasis also appears to be associated with few or no manifestations of disease in individuals examined in field environments. In a controlled study involving clinical examination, evaluation of growth and development, hematological studies, and screening tests for intestinal malabsorption, no significant differences between positive and negative subjects were found [9]. Cases of severe clinical illness characterized by diarrhea, abdominal pain, edema (often facial), and passage of undigested food in the feces have been reported. In most of these cases, worm burdens appear to have been very heavy [9].

Paragonimiasis usually comes to the attention of the physician when the patient complains of cough [10]. Another important finding is a history of intermittent hemoptysis. Profuse expectoration and chest pain of a pleuritic type are also frequently found in symptomatic patients. Nevertheless, surveys and clinical studies of groups of individuals indicate that in most endemic areas the majority of infections due to *Paragonimus* are light or moderate and are associated with few signs or symptoms [10]. Cerebral paragonimiasis is encountered in highly endemic regions and appears to occur largely in those persons who are heavily infected after the onset of pulmonary symptoms. The clinical signs and symptoms are similar to those of Jacksonian epilepsy, cerebral tumors, or embolism of the brain [10].

Diagnosis

The progression to a diagnosis of fluke infection is shown in figure 1. The anatomical location of the symptoms and signs will provide an obvious means of deciding whether there is a possibility of liver, intestinal, or lung fluke infection. Except in the case of fascioliasis, the geographic history should be of particular value, as all of the other fluke infections of humans are found largely in Asia. A careful dietary history is of great importance and will provide a relatively clear-cut decision, as consumption of aquatic vegetation, raw fish, or raw crustacea is essential to establishment of the infection.

A definitive diagnosis will be provided by demonstration of the eggs of the parasite in the feces in all cases of hermaphroditic fluke infection, although eggs are also found in the sputum of persons with paragonimiasis. As the characteristic ova are often scanty in the feces, a concentration procedure is necessary; the best method is the formol-ether technique. With use of applicator sticks, mix approximately 2 ml of feces into a 15-ml centrifuge tube half full of saline. Add saline to within one-half inch of the top and mix again. Centrifuge for 1 min at 1,000 *g*, decant (sediment should be about 1 ml), resuspend in saline, centrifuge, and decant. Add 10% buffered formalin to the sediment until the tube is half full, mix, and allow to stand for 5 min. Add 3 ml of ether, shake vigorously, and centrifuge at 600 *g* for 2 min. Ring the tube with an applicator stick, and carefully decant the top three layers, leaving the sediment. With the applicator sticks, remove the sediment onto a slide, add a drop of iodine stain and a cover slip, and examine under the microscope. Eggs of *Fasciola, Fasciolopsis,* and *Paragonimus* are large and will be easily seen at ×100 magnification. For examination of sputum, the specimen should be treated with 3% NaOH to dissolve the mucus and then centrifuged. The sediment should be examined under the microscope.

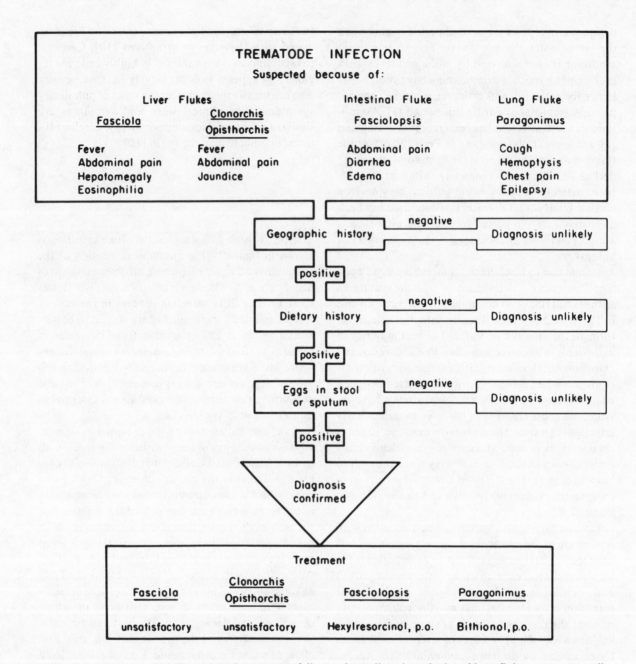

Figure 1. Progression to the diagnosis and treatment of disease due to liver, intestinal, and lung flukes; p.o. = perorally.

Chest X-rays of persons with paragonimiasis are not characteristic and often are similar to those taken of persons with pulmonary tuberculosis. In cerebral paragonimiasis, X-rays of the brain reveal calcification in approximately half of the cases.

Management

The proper treatment of fascioliasis in man has been

exceedingly difficult to establish because of the sporadic nature of the infection, and presumably self-limited clinical syndrome, and the apparent necessity for prolonged treatment with potentially toxic drugs such as emetine and chloroquine. Long-term, careful follow-up study reveals that many cases are not cured [1]. Steroids should not be used because they have been shown to exacerbate pathological changes in experimental animals. Since a drug regimen of proven value has not been established for clonorchiasis and opisthorchiasis, it is fortunate that treatment is not required in the majority of cases. Surgery, relieving blockage of the bile duct systems, may be necessary in the treatment of cholangitis. For fasciolopsiasis, hexylresorcinol in a single oral dose of 1 g is the treatment of choice, and for paragonimiasis, bithionol is given orally in a dose of 30 mg/kg on alternate days for a total of 10 doses. Skin reactions and gastrointestinal irritation have been reported but are rarely severe enough to interrupt treatment. (Both hexylresorcinol and bithionol may be obtained from the Parasitic Diseases Branch, Center for Disease Control, Atlanta, Ga. 30333.)

References

1. Facey, R. V., Marsden, P. D. Fascioliasis in man: an outbreak in Hampshire. Br. Med. J. 2:619–625, 1960.
2. Hardman, E. W., Jones, R. L. H., Davies, A. H. Fascioliasis—a large outbreak. Br. Med. J. 3:502–505, 1970.
3. Stork, M. G., Venables, G. S., Jennings, S. M. F., Beesley, J. R., Bendezu, P., Capron, A. An investigation of endemic fascioliasis in Peruvian village children. J. Trop. Med. Hyg. 76:231–235, 1973.
4. Strauss, W. G. Clinical manifestations of clonorchiasis. A controlled study of 105 cases. Am. J. Trop. Med. Hyg. 11:625–630, 1962.
5. Choi, D. W., Kim, J. W., Park, S. B. Laboratory findings in symptomless clonorchiasis. Korean J. Parasitol. 8:8–12, 1970.
6. Wykoff, D. E., Chittayasothorn, K., Winn, N. M. Clinical manifestations of *Opisthorchis viverrini* infections in Thailand. Am. J. Trop. Med. Hyg. 15:914–918, 1966.
7. Fung, J. Liver fluke infestation and cholangio-hepatitis. Br. J. Surg. 48:404–415, 1961.
8. Viranuvatti, V., Stitnimankarn, T. Liver fluke infection and infestation in Southeast Asia. *In* H. Popper and F. Schaffner [ed.]. Progress in liver diseases. Vol. 4. Grune and Stratton, New York, 1972, p. 537–547.
9. Plaut, A. G., Kamapanart-Sanyakorn, C., Manning, G. S. A clinical study of *Fasciolopsis buski* infection in Thailand. Trans. R. Soc. Trop. Med. Hyg. 63:470–478, 1969.
10. Yokogawa, S., Cort, W. W., Yokogawa, M. Paragonimus and paragonimiasis. Exp. Parasitol. 10:139–205, 1960.

Hookworm

Two species of hookworm (*Ancylostoma duodenale* and *Necator americanus*) are major human helminthic parasites. These organisms directly penetrate the skin and migrate through the lungs to reach their final habitat in the small intestine, where they adhere to the intestinal mucosa and ingest blood. In heavy infections blood loss may be sufficient to produce iron deficiency anemia. Although the hookworms have a relatively low endemicity in the United States (largely in the southeast), an estimated one-fourth of the world's population is infected [1]. Transient visitors to endemic areas are likely to acquire only light, asymptomatic infections, but long-term residents or immigrants, particularly from rural areas, may develop significant infections that require treatment.

Life Cycle

The life cycles of the two types of hookworm that infect humans, *A. duodenale* and *N. americanus,* are similar [2]. Larvae hatch from eggs in feces deposited onto soil. After two molts, the larvae are infective for humans and are able to penetrate the skin. Contact with contaminated soil for 5–10 min is required for skin penetration; such contact may occur when people walk barefoot, handle soil bare-handed, or ingest soil. The larvae are then conducted by the circulatory system to the lungs, make their way through the alveolar walls to the bronchi and trachea, and are carried with swallowed secretions to their final habitat in the small intestine. Two further molts occur in the intestine before the parasites reach maturity and start egg production (four to six weeks after skin penetration).

The adult worms are grayish-white and slightly curved and measure 5–13 mm in length. In spite of the name *A. duodenale,* hookworms are found largely in the jejunum, where they attach to the mucosa by tooth-like structures in their buccal cavities. Blood and mucosal substances are ingested, and much of this

material is excreted. The average blood loss and egg output in *A. duodenale* infections (0.15 ml of blood per worm per day; 25,000 eggs per worm per day) are several times greater than in *N. americanus* infections (0.03 ml of blood per worm per day; 7,000 eggs per worm per day) [2, 3]. Hookworms do not multiply within the human host, and the average life-span of *N. americanus* adults is reportedly two to six years. The survival time for *A. duodenale* is supposedly shorter, but satisfactory data on mean life-span are not available [3].

Epidemiology

Although earlier reports described distinct distributions, both *A. duodenale* and *N. americanus* are found in most regions of the world. Hookworms are especially common in the agrarian tropical areas of Africa, Asia, Central and South America, and the Caribbean countries, where conditions for the development and survival of larvae are optimal: well-aerated, moderately moist, shaded soil with temperatures between 23°C and 33°C [2]. This environment also exists in the southeastern United States, where 42% of white inhabitants had *N. americanus* infections in the early 20th century [4]. The pioneering work of the Rockefeller Sanitary Commission in the decade between 1910 and 1920 substantially reduced the incidence of hookworm infection in the United States. At present, the prevalence of infection ranges from 2% to 15% among children and young adults in some rural southern areas; infections are usually light and asymptomatic [4].

Disease Syndromes

Although hookworm infection exists with the establishment of a single hookworm in the body, hookworm disease occurs only when infection is heavy enough to result in clinical manifestations. The majority of people with hookworm have light infections without disease. For instance, in Venezuela 726 of 796 individuals (91%) with *N. americanus* infections had low egg counts and no anemia. Only egg counts of >2,000/ml of feces in women and children or >5,000/ml of feces in men were associated with anemia [3].

The major manifestations of hookworm disease are iron deficiency anemia and hypoalbuminemia; these conditions result from chronic gastrointestinal blood loss. Blood loss is proportional to the number of hookworms present; the worm burden depends on the number of larvae that successfully penetrate the skin and the life-span of the worms. The observed blood loss can be accounted for entirely by the ingestion of blood by hookworms [3]. Hematologic status reflects the balance between iron lost from the gastrointestinal tract and iron absorbed from dietary sources. Thus, the worm burden at which anemia appears depends on the amount of absorbable dietary iron. Populations whose major foods are deficient in iron or inhibit iron absorption [3] develop anemia at lower egg counts than those with readily available and absorbable dietary iron. Similarly, in individual cases the worm burden may not accurately predict anemia because of variation in iron intake.

Acute infection. Primary skin penetration by larvae is associated with little reaction, but multiple exposures may result in "ground itch"—intense pruritis, edema, erythema, and a papulo-vesicular rash in the area of larval entry. The migration of larvae through the lungs usually causes few or no symptoms, but in some cases cough with bloody eosinophil-containing sputum, dyspnea, and a peripheral eosinophilia may develop about a week after skin penetration [2]. In experimental infections with massive inocula (400 *A. duodenale* larvae in one dose), the phase of attachment to the small intestinal mucosa was associated with several weeks of abdominal pain, diarrhea, and weight loss; these symptoms disappeared as the larvae matured and the condition became chronic. There have been no adequate studies of gastrointestinal symptoms in naturally occurring infections.

Chronic infection. The only clinically significant consequences of chronic heavy hookworm infection are iron deficiency anemia and occasional hypoalbuminemia. The iron deficiency anemia of hookworm disease is indistinguishable from that of chronic blood loss due to other causes, and few symptoms are present until anemia is moderate or severe. As the hemoglobin level falls, patients may complain of fatigability, headache, numbness and tingling, dyspnea, palpitations, anorexia, dyspepsia, pedal edema, and sexual dysfunction. In children there may be growth failure, irritability, behavior problems, and impaired intellectual functioning.

Physical findings are present in hookworm disease only if there is significant anemia; these symptoms include pallor, tachycardia, increased precordial activity, systolic murmurs, slight hepatosplenomegaly, and dependent edema. Gastrointestinal protein loss may contribute to edema formation. In the absence of preexisting cardiac or pulmonary disease, cardiac decompensation, which may be fatal, rarely occurs before the hemoglobin level is < 6 g/100 ml.

Anemia and iron deficiency are the only consistent laboratory findings; occult blood is often found in the stool, and in severe cases the level of serum albumin may be low. In children malabsorption has been reported and is similar to that found in iron deficiency anemia of other causes. In adults clinical malabsorption has been reported only rarely; mild nonspecific abnormalities occasionally seen on X-rays of the bowel or intestinal biopsies are usually unaccompanied by symptoms [3].

Diagnosis

The process of diagnosis and management of hookworm infection and disease in a nonendemic area is illustrated in the accompanying algorithm (figure 1). The patient is most likely to present with the signs and symptoms of iron deficiency anemia. A history of residence or travel in an endemic area and skin contact with contaminated soil should cause the physician to consider the diagnosis of hookworm disease. People who always wear shoes, use latrines, and do not handle soil are unlikely to harbor hookworms and certainly would not harbor a clinically significant number. The patient's report of "ground itch," cough, and transient gastrointestinal distress are suggestive but not diagnostic of hookworm disease. Except under experimental conditions diagnosis of hookworm infection during larval migration through the skin, lungs, and gastrointestinal tract is not possible because mature, egg-producing adults are not yet present.

The eggs of *A. duodenale* and *N. americanus* are indistinguishable. Identification by species is possible only through examination of larvae after egg culture or of adult worms after treatment. Such procedures are rarely necessary in the treatment of an individual patient. Initial screening for eggs is done by direct fecal smear. A drop of iodine solution (1% potassium iodide saturated with iodine) and a small amount of feces are mixed on a slide with an applicator stick, covered, and examined under low power. Since the egg output per worm is very high, direct smear is adequate for the diagnosis of clinically significant hookworm infection. This technique will identify egg

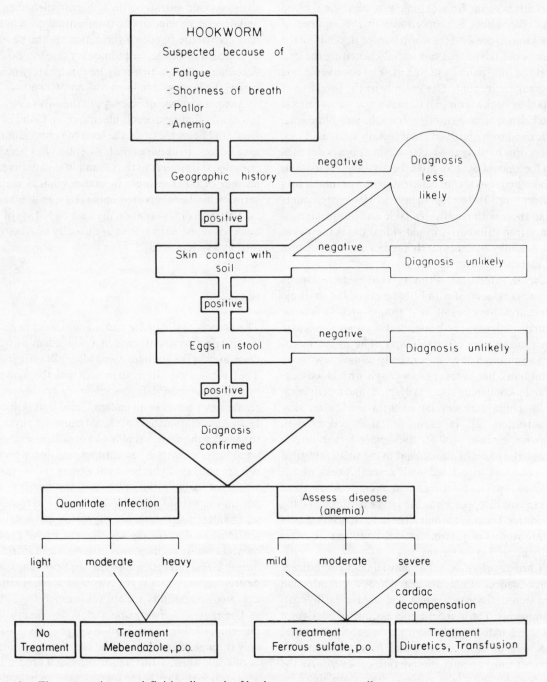

Figure 1.   The progression to a definitive diagnosis of hookworm; p.o. = perorally.

counts of > 1,200 eggs/ml [2], a level well below those associated with anemia; thus it is not necessary to concentrate the feces.

While the diagnosis of hookworm infection is established by simple demonstration of hookworm eggs in the patient's feces, the diagnosis of hookworm disease requires documentation of a significant worm burden by quantitative egg counts. Egg counts of > 2,000/ml of feces in women and children or > 5,000/ml in men are associated with anemia in Venezuela [3], a country in which iron is likely to be less available than in the United States. Although the Venezuelan studies involved *N. americanus* infections, the counts are applicable to *A. duodenale* because the greater blood loss caused by this parasite is compensated for by its greater egg output. Egg counts higher than those mentioned above suggest that an associated anemia is due to hookworm disease, but other common causes of anemia should be sought.

Positive direct smear is followed, therefore, by quantitative techniques that involve dilution of the stool because of the high output of eggs by the hookworms. The modified Stoll method, in which a known volume of stool rather than a known weight is used, is simplest [5]. (*1*) A Stoll flask (available from Arthur H. Thomas, Philadelphia, Pa.) is filled to the 56-ml mark with 0.1 N sodium hydroxide (4 g of sodium hydroxide crystals dissolved in distilled water added to make 1,000 ml); feces are added until the fluid level reaches the 60-ml mark. (*2*) About eight glass beads (approximately 6 mm in diameter) are added, the flask is closed with a rubber stopper, it is shaken vigorously with an up-and-down motion for 60 sec, and the solution is set aside until the next morning. (*3*) The flask is shaken again, and 0.15 ml of solution is withdrawn immediately, placed on a 3- × 2-inch slide, and covered with a 22- × 40-mm coverslip. (*4*) All eggs on the slide are counted under low power by systematic scanning of the preparation. (*5*) The number of eggs is multiplied by 100 to obtain the number of eggs per ml of formed feces (for soft ' stools the product is multiplied by 2, for watery stools by 4).

Management

Most hookworm infections require no treatment, since they are light and are not associated with disease. Moderate to heavy infections that are capable of producing anemia should be recognized and treated.

The treatment of individual cases of hookworm disease is best accomplished with mebendazole (Vermox,® Ortho Pharmaceutical Corp., Raritan, N.J.), a broad-spectrum oral anthelmintic agent that is poorly absorbed and has few side effects [6]. The dose is 100 mg twice a day for three days regardless of the patient's body weight. With this regimen 95% of *N. americanus* infections are cured, and egg counts are reduced by 99.9% in the remaining cases. Initial

studies with *A. duodenale* have shown a similarly favorable response. Eradication of the infection is not mandatory, since small numbers of hookworms are not associated with disease. None of the drugs commonly used in the treatment of hookworm (mebendazole, bephenium hydroxynaphthoate, tetrachloroethylene, and pyrantel pamoate) is recommended for use during pregnancy. The infected pregnant woman should be treated for iron deficiency anemia and mebendazole use postponed until after delivery. Transmission by infected individuals is not a significant problem in the United States (except in parts of the rural south), since the use of shoes and latrines virtually prevents the spread of this parasite.

Anthelmintics alone will produce hematologic improvement, but correction of anemia may be slow without supplementation of dietary iron. Conversely, iron therapy will raise the hemoglobin level without anthelmintic drugs, but anemia may recur unless the hookworm infection is treated. Therefore, the management of hookworm disease requires both reduction of worm burden and iron therapy. Oral iron is well absorbed even in severe cases. The dose for adults is 60 mg of elemental ferrous iron (300 mg of ferrous sulfate) given between meals three times a day. For children 2 mg of elemental iron/kg per dose is administered orally on a similar schedule. Where anemia is so severe as to threaten life and there are signs of heart failure, a diuretic should be administered and followed by slow transfusion with packed red blood cells.

References

1. Davis, A. Drug treatment in intestinal helminthiasis. World Health Organization, Geneva, 1973, p. 52–89.
2. Belding, D. L. Textbook of parasitology. 3rd ed. Appleton-Century-Crofts, New York, 1965, p. 423–447.
3. Roche, M., Layrisse, M. The nature and causes of "hookworm anemia" Am. J. Trop. Med. Hyg. 15:1030–1100, 1966.
4. Warren, K. S. Helminthic diseases endemic in the United States. Am. J. Trop. Med. Hyg. 23:723–730, 1974.
5. Melvin, D. M., Brooke, M. M. Laboratory procedures for the diagnosis of intestinal parasites. U.S. Department of Health, Education and Welfare (publication no. [CDC] 75-8282), Atlanta, Ga., 1974, p. 158–162.
6. Mebendazole—a new anthelmintic. Med. Lett. Drugs Ther. 17:37–38, 1975.

Schistosomiasis

Schistosomiasis is a chronic helminth infection, caused by three different species of blood flukes— *Schistosoma mansoni, S. japonicum* and *S. haematobium*—which afflicts more than 200 million people in Asia, Africa, the Caribbean and South America. Man is infected on entry into contaminated fresh water by direct skin penetration of larvae emitted by the snail intermediate hosts. The young parasites (schistosomula) migrate from the skin to the lungs and through the liver to the final habitats of the adult worms in the venules of the intestines (*S. mansoni* and *S. japonicum*) or urinary bladder (*S. haematobium*). Since the schistosomes do not multiply within the definitive mammalian host, many individuals harbor relatively low worm burdens. Disease appears to be associated with intensity of infection and is due to the deposition of large numbers of parasite eggs in the host tissues, not only of the intestines and urinary bladder, but of the liver, lungs, ureters and even the central nervous system.

The most common severe disease manifestations are related to the host inflammatory and fibrotic response to the eggs in the liver resulting in obstruction to portal blood flow and hepatosplenic disease, the lungs leading to blockage of pulmonary blood flow and cardiopulmonary disease, and the ureters impeding urine flow and culminating in hydronephrosis.

Although the lack of suitable snail intermediate hosts precludes the transmission of schistosomiasis in the continental United States, it has been estimated that one-tenth of the 1.5 million resident Puerto Rican population had this chronic infection when they entered the country [1]. In addition, some 100,000 individuals from other areas of the world that are endemic for schistosomiasis (principally the Philippines, but also the West Indies, Africa, and Brazil) migrate to America each year. Two other factors have also contributed to the presence of infected individuals in the United States: international jet travel, which has led to exposure of increasing numbers of tourists and businessmen, and the return of American troops from their deployment in endemic areas of the world. Thus the number of infected persons in the continental United States has become and will continue to be a diagnostic and therapeutic problem with which the American physician should be more familiar. Furthermore, the drugs available for treatment are potentially toxic, and should be applied judiciously and with care.

Life Cycle

Although there are many species of mammalian and avian schistosomes, three major species develop to maturity in man: *S. mansoni, S. japonicum,* and *S. haematobium.* Each of these organisms has a different geographic distribution: *S. mansoni* occurs in Arabia, Africa, South America, and the Caribbean; *S. japonicum* in Japan, China, and the Philippines; and *S. haematobium* in Africa and the Middle East. The adult schistosomes are trematode flukes of both sexes that reside in the mesenteric and vesical venules of man. The male and female worms are approximately 1–2 cm long, and the female lies within a cleft in the body of the male worm. The female worm produces large numbers of eggs (300–3,000 per day per worm pair). Through the combined action of enzymatic secretions and peristalsis, these eggs pass out of the blood vessels, through the tissues, and into the lumen of the gut (*S. mansoni* and *S. japonicum*) or the urinary bladder (*S. haematobium*), leaving the body via the feces or urine.

On reaching fresh water the eggs hatch into ciliated miracidia, which must find and penetrate into a specific species of snail in order to multiply and continue their development. (It is the absence of these particular species of snails that prevents the human schistosomes from completing their life cycles in the continental United States.) Within the snail, one miracidium may develop into hundreds or thousands of cercariae, the infective form for both avian and mammalian species. Large numbers of free-swimming cercariae may emerge from the snails daily. On coming into contact with human skin, they can penetrate rapidly (within 3–10 min for *S. mansoni* and as quickly as 30 sec for *S. japonicum*). Once in the body, the young schistosomes migrate to the lungs and then to the hepatoportal system, where they mature, mate, and pass down into the mesenteric or vesical venules to begin production of eggs. When schistosomes that cannot live in a human host attack man, the cercariae die in the skin.

Epidemiology

An important characteristic that distinguishes schistosomes and most other helminth parasites from virtually all other infectious agents is that the adult worms do not multiply in the human body. This fact has profound implications with respect to the pathogenesis, clinical appearance, and therapeutic aspects of helminth infections. Under these conditions, the major factors governing worm burdens in infected individuals are the rate of acquisition of new worms and the life-span of the worms already present in the body. Recent studies in endemic areas suggest that the level of infectivity in most bodies of fresh water is relatively low, because few snails are infected and cercariae are dispersed in large volumes of water [2]. The rate of uptake of worms, therefore, is usually low, and brief contact with contaminated water is rarely associated with significant infection. Only occasionally are individuals exposed to conditions in which cercarial density is high; these persons may acquire heavy worm burdens. While we know that each of the three species of schistosome that infect humans is capable of living for 20–30 years in its human host, recent figures suggest that the mean life-span of *S. mansoni* is probably between five and 10 years [3]. Moreover, studies of the relationship between worm burden and the development of significant pathology in the human definitive host reveal that light infections appear to have few clinical consequences and that disease is found mainly in patients with large worm loads, who constitute only a small proportion of the infected populations [4–6].

Disease Syndromes

Three major disease syndromes occur in schistosomiasis: schistosome dermatitis, acute schistosomiasis, and chronic schistosomiasis.

(1) Schistosome dermatitis. It is unlikely that this problem will be seen in the United States in association with infection by schistosomes in humans, because dermatitis appears within 24 hr after penetration of the cercariae into the skin and disappears within a few days. This reaction which occurs only after repeated exposure appears to be an immunological response with both immediate and delayed components [7]. Schistosomes that infect birds and animals are ubiquitous, however, and the allergic reaction produced when their cercariae die in attempting to penetrate human skin may be encountered. This problem is common in the region of the Great Lakes of the north-central United States and has been reported from many other parts of the country, including those in which brackish and salt as well as fresh waters are found. Except for the occasional severe case, this manifestation of schistosomiasis is mainly a nuisance. It must be kept in mind, however, that all schistosomes cross-react in many immunological tests used for diagnosis. Thus 26% of individuals skin-tested with *S. mansoni* antigen in northern Michigan had positive reactions [8].

(2) Acute schistosomiasis (Katayama fever). This syndrome will rarely be seen in the United States, since it seems to occur only during primary infection in individuals exposed to high cercarial concentrations and has many characteristics in common with antigen–antibody complex mediated serum sickness [7]. Katayama fever begins between four and eight weeks after exposure and lasts for just a few weeks. It appears most commonly in *S. japonicum* infection, is much less common in *S. mansoni* infections, and is seen quite rarely in patients with schistosomiasis haematobia. This disease state is characterized by an acute febrile illness, cough, hepatosplenomegaly, lymphadenopathy, and eosinophilia. Although Katayama fever is self-limited and disappears within several weeks, it can result in severe morbidity and even death, particularly in heavy *S. japonicum* infections.

(3) Chronic schistosomiasis. This is the stage of infection during which most patients in the United States will be seen and at which the physician should be able to identify and diagnose schistosomiasis. Although a wide variety of symptoms has been associated with chronic schistosomiasis (including fatigue, abdominal pain, and intermittent diarrhea or dysentery in *S. japonicum* and *S. mansoni* infection, and dysuria in *S. haematobium* infection), recent field studies of schistosomiasis mansoni have demonstrated few specific symptoms, whether the patients have light or heavy infections [3, 5, 6]. However, in a proportion of patients (usually those with heavy worm

loads), the chronic stage may eventually reveal itself by the development of significant disease.

While approximately 40% of the schistosome eggs pass out of the body and continue the life cycle, the remaining 60% either remain in the local tissues or pass via the bloodstream into the next organ system, in which they are trapped as the veins decrease in caliber. These eggs elicit a marked granulomatous reaction by the host which is an immunological response of the delayed hypersensitivity type and results in considerable destruction of tissue and fibrosis [7]. With respect to the pathogenesis of hepatosplenic disease, the eggs themselves appear to cause little significant obstruction of blood flow, but the granulomatous and fibrotic response of the host creates an intrahepatic presinusoidal block, leading to portal hypertension and esophageal varices. The liver parenchymal cells are not directly harmed by the disease process; furthermore, arterial neovascular formation maintains total hepatic blood flow within normal limits, providing adequate hepatocyte perfusion. Thus results of tests of hepatic function are usually normal, and there are few if any of the stigmata of chronic hepatic disease.

Clinically, the earliest sign of involvement of the liver is hepatomegaly, which may be followed by the development of an enlarged, firm spleen. The major complication of hepatosplenic schistosomiasis is the occurrence of bleeding esophageal varices, as manifested by hematemesis, but the consequences of this condition are far different from those in patients with cirrhosis of the liver. The mortality rate resulting from a hematemesis in cirrhosis is at least 60%, but the death rate in schistosomiasis is low because most patients have well-functioning livers and do not develop hepatic coma. Hematemesis may recur often in some patients, but in others there may be years between episodes. While individuals with schistosomiasis may also develop signs and symptoms related to liver parenchymal damage (including jaundice, ascites, and stigmata of liver disease), it is not known whether this is a natural progression of the schistosome infection or is related to additional factors, such as hepatitis.

Since few immigrants are from areas endemic for schistosomiasis haematobia, chronic urinary tract disease will rarely be seen. The major cause of disease is obstruction to urine flow as a result of florid granuloma formation around masses of *S. haematobium* eggs and subsequent fibrosis. This condition may lead to hydronephrosis and, eventually, uremia. Symptoms may also be related to reduced distensibility of the bladder because of calcification of the eggs and fibrosis. The incidence of cancer of the bladder is increased in schistosomiasis haematobia.

Other aspects of chronic schistosomiasis should be mentioned, although it is unlikely that they will be encountered by physicians in the United States. Polyps, the major complication of intestinal disease, are seen almost exclusively in Egypt. Patients with severe hepatosplenic schistosomiasis and portal systemic collateral circulation may develop pulmonary involvement as a result of bypass of the liver by eggs, which are then sieved out in the lungs. Granuloma formation around the eggs and arteritis obstruct blood flow, leading to pulmonary hypertension and cor pulmonale. Involvement of the central nervous system, although rare, is a complication of major importance, the etiology of which appears to be the large masses of eggs laid by ectopic worm pairs. *S. japonicum* tends to localize within the brain and is associated with the development of focal epilepsy or diffuse cerebral disease, while *S. mansoni* and *S. haematobium* are usually found in the spinal cord and are associated with a transverse myelitis-like syndrome.

Diagnosis

To facilitate the diagnosis and management of schistosomiasis in a nonendemic area, we have prepared an algorithm, or flow sheet, in which a progression to a definitive diagnosis is made through a series of logical steps (figure 1). The key to this approach is the physician's suspicion that his patient has schistosomiasis. The patient may actually suggest the diagnosis, or there may be marked eosinophilia, indicating the presence of a helminth infection; in schistosomiasis mansoni and japonica the patient may appear with hepatosplenomegaly or, in the most extreme case, have a hematemesis; in *S. haematobium* infection, hematuria and dysuria would suggest the diagnosis.

Once schistosomiasis is suspected, a geographic history must be obtained, since distribution of the various schistosome species is well defined (table 1), and a negative history of exposure to sites where the disease might be acquired would rule out the diagnosis. If the geographic history is positive, the next step is the establishment of whether or not there has been significant contact with fresh water within an

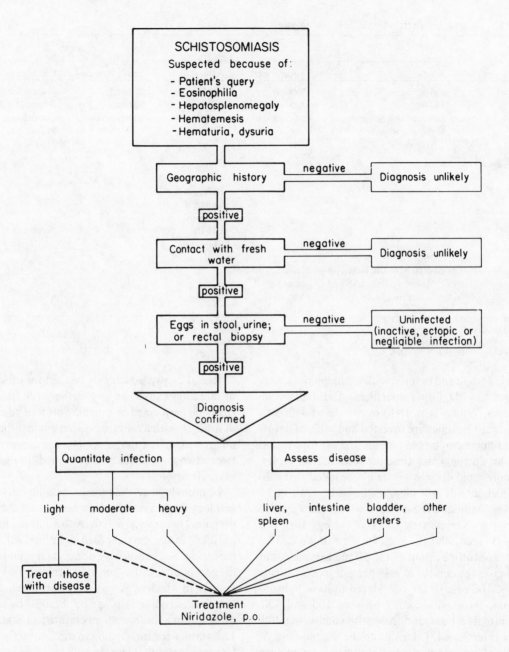

Figure 1. The progression to a definitive diagnosis of schistosomiasis; p.o. = perorally.

endemic area. Schistosomiasis in humans is essentially not transmissible in salt water, adequate chlorination of fresh water obviates infection, and it is unlikely that a chance momentary exposure (such as being splashed with water or wading rapidly across a stream) would result in infection.

If both the geographic history and the history of water contact are positive, a definitive diagnosis can then be made by demonstration of eggs in the patient's feces or urine or by rectal biopsy. The Kato thick smear is the procedure of choice at present for determination of eggs in the feces. The test is simple to perform and provides not only qualitative but also quantitative information. Since schistosome eggs are distributed randomly in a sample of feces, only a small portion is needed for the test. A 50-mg sample of feces that has been pressed through 105-mesh stainless steel bolting cloth (W. S. Tyler, Cleveland, Ohio) is placed

Table 1. Geographic distribution of schistosomiasis.

Species of Schistosoma	Area				
	Africa	Middle East	Asia	South America	Caribbean
mansoni	Egypt	Yemen		Brazil	Puerto Rico
	Sudan	Arabia		Surinam	Dominican Republic†
	South of the Sahara*			Venezuela	Guadeloupe
	Malagasy Republic				Martinique
					St. Lucia
japonicum			China		
			Japan		
			Philippines		
			Celebes†		
			Thailand†		
			Laos†		
			Cambodia†		
haematobium	Everywhere (including	Iran†			
	Malagasy Republic and	Iraq			
	Mauritius)	Yemen			
		Arabia			

  * Focal distribution.
  † Very small focal areas.

on a glass slide and covered with a cellophane cover-slip (no. 124 PD, Film Department, E. I. DuPont de Nemours, Wilmington, Del.) impregnated with 50% glycerine. The slides are inverted and pressed onto a bed of filter paper, turned face up, and left for a period of 48 hr. during which time the fecal matter clears. For more rapid diagnosis it should be noted that a 20 mg fecal sample will clear and can be read in 15 minutes. Although the embryo within the egg also clears, the characteristic shape of the egg shell can easily be seen, and the eggs in the sample can be counted. Multiplication of the 50 mg sample count by 20 gives the number of eggs per g of feces. Patients with < 100 eggs/g are considered to have light infections, those with counts between 100 and 400, moderate infections, and those with counts over 400, heavy infections [5]. Urine for the diagnosis of S. haematobium infection is best collected between noon and 2 P.M. The presence of eggs can easily be ascertained by scanning of the lightly centrifuged sediment. Counts can be made by passing a 10-ml aliquot of the urine sample through a Nuclepore filter (13 mm in diameter with a pore size of 8 μm) held in a PT-103 chamber (Nuclepore Corp., Pleasanton, California). The filter is removed, placed face down on a microscope slide and examined immediately at ×40 magnification. The terminal spined eggs can be clearly seen [9].

Rectal biopsy, which may be used for the diagnosis of infection caused by any of the three species, can easily be performed by pinching off four small pieces of mucosa with a curette pressed against the edge of an anoscope. The tissue samples are compressed between two glass slides and examined for eggs at low magnification.

Immunological diagnostic techniques, such as serology or skin tests, cannot be used for a definitive diagnosis because of reactivity to human schistosome antigens in patients exposed to animal schistosome cercariae. Such tests may be necessary, however, for diagnosis of schistosomiasis of the central nervous system, in which eggs may not be present in the feces or urine. Serodiagnosis can be obtained by sending 1 ml of serum at ambient temperature to a State Health Laboratory for forwarding to the Center for Disease Control, Atlanta, Georgia.

If the patient presents with hepatic disease, its relation to schistosome infection can be established by demonstration of hepatosplenomegaly and portal systemic collateral circulation in the presence of relatively normal liver parenchymal function. A major differential diagnosis is portal vein thrombosis, which can be ruled out by splenoportography. Involvement of the urinary tract in schistosomiasis haematobia can be determined by iv pyelography and, when necessary, retrograde pyelography and cystoscopy.

Management

Certain aspects of the host-parasite relationship in schistosomiasis help to delineate the basic objectives of therapy. The worms do not multiply in the human host, they have a relatively limited life-span, and light infections appear to be of little pathological significance, except in rare cases in which the central nervous system is involved. Furthermore, the only drugs available for treatment are toxic and do not always provide a parasitological cure. An additional factor is that patients seen in the United States cannot be reinfected and do not constitute a public health hazard. Thus the aim of treatment might well be to reduce the worm burden rather than to attempt a parasitological cure, which would require high doses of drugs. Treatment is recommended, therefore, for patients with moderate and heavy infections, and for those with light infections if they have signs and symptoms of disease.

Niridazole is the drug of choice, since it is both reasonably effective and safe. The drug can be obtained from the Parasitic Drug Service of the Center for Disease Control in Atlanta, Ga. Niridazole is administered orally in divided daily doses of 25 mg/kg of body weight (maximum, 1,500 mg) per day for seven days. Loss of appetite, nausea, insomnia, vomiting, dizziness, and slight changes in hepatic enzymes or electrocardiogram may occur, but in most cases these side effects will not interfere with completion of the course of therapy. The drug should be administered under strict medical supervision, preferably in a hospital. Its use is contraindicated in patients with hepatic, cerebral, or psychotic diseases. Under these circumstances, antimony dimercaptosuccinate (stibocaptate) may be used; it also is available from the Parasitic Drug Service. It is administered biweekly or weekly in im injections of 250 mg, with a total of eight doses. The side effects of stibocaptate are similar to those of niridazole, but since the former is an antimonial compound, its cardiac toxicity tends to be more severe, and the drug may be lethal.

Recently, the technique of extracorporeal hemofiltration has been recommended as a means of therapy; by a combination of surgery and a single dose of antischistosomal drug, the worms are sieved out of the bloodstream. This technique is largely of academic interest and should never be used in the treatment of schistosomiasis.

In addition to specific antischistosomal therapy, some patients with the sequelae of chronic fibroobstructive lesions may need further medical attention. Most important is the patient with hepatosplenomegaly and bleeding esophageal varices. Conservative treatment along general medical lines is the best policy, and surgical interference should be used only as a last resort if the patient has repeated episodes of bleeding. Since portocaval shunts are associated with an unacceptable degree of chronic portal systemic encephalopathy, splenorenal anastomosis with its much smaller stoma is now considered to be the preferable operation. For schistosomiasis haematobia, procedures that restore the patency of the ureteral-vesical junction must occasionally be used, but only if medical treatment yields no significant change in the state of the patient.

References

1. Warren, K. S. Helminthic diseases endemic in the United States. Am. J. Trop. Med. Hyg. 23:723–730, 1974.
2. Warren, K. S. Regulation of the prevalence and intensity of schistosomiasis in man: immunology or ecology? J. Infect. Dis. 127:595–609, 1973.
3. Warren, K. S., Mahmoud, A. A. F., Cummings, P., Murphy, D. J., Houser, H. B. Schistosomiasis mansoni in Yemeni in California: duration of infection, presence of disease, therapeutic management. Am. J. Trop. Med. Hyg. 23:902–909, 1974.
4. Cheever, A. W. A quantitative post-mortem study of schistosomiasis mansoni in man. Am. J. Trop. Med. Hyg. 17:38–64, 1968.
5. Arap Siongok, T. K., Mahmoud, A. A. F., Ouma, J. H., Warren, K. S., Muller, A. S., Handa, A. K., Houser, H. B. Morbidity in schistosomiasis mansoni in relation to intensity of infection: Study of a community in Machakos, Kenya. Am. J. Trop. Med. Hyg. 25:273–284, 1976.
6. Lehman, J. S., Jr., Mott, K. E., Morrow, R. H., Jr., Muniz, T. M., Boyer, M. H. The intensity and effects of infection with *Schistosoma mansoni* in a rural community in Northeast Brazil. Am. J. Trop. Med. Hyg. 25:285–294, 1976.
7. Warren, K. S. Schistosomiasis: a multiplicity of immunopathology. J. Invest. Dermatol. 67:464–468, 1976.
8. Moore, G. T., Kaiser, R. C., Lawrence, R. S., Putnam, S. M., Kagan, I. G. Intradermal and serologic reactions to antigens from *Schistosoma mansoni* in schistosome dermatitis. Am. J. Trop. Med. Hyg. 17:86–91, 1968.
9. Peters, P. A., Mahmoud, A. A. F., Warren, K. S., Ouma, J. H., Arap Siongok, T. K. Field studies of a rapid, accurate means of quantifying *Schistosoma haematobium* eggs in urine samples. Bull. World Health Org. 54:159–162, 1976.

Strongyloidiasis

Strongyloidiasis is a potentially lethal helminth infection for which effective treatment is now available. Unlike most other helminth parasites, which do not multiply within man, *Strongyloides stercoralis* has the capacity to cause an overwhelming infection via a process called autoinfection. The incidence of this complication appears to be markedly enhanced in immunodepressed individuals.

S. stercoralis, although uncommon in comparison with the other major intestinal nematodes, is widely distributed through the tropics and has a patchy distribution in temperate regions. In the United States, surveys from the southern and border states indicate a prevalence of 0.4%–4%. Occasional autochthonous cases have been found in northern cities. Prevalence in institutions, particularly those for the intellectually retarded, may be high, with 5%–35% of the inmates infected. Imported cases are seen most often in immigrants from Puerto Rico and other areas of the Caribbean and in veterans of wars in Southeast Asia.

Life Cycle

Although man is the principal host of *S. stercoralis,* the parasite can survive and reproduce in the soil. There are three possible cycles.

(1) The free-living cycle. The basic life cycle of the parasite takes place in water-logged topsoil. Larvae passed in the feces from an infected host moult and differentiate into free-living males and females. After fertilization, eggs are released and hatch into rhabditiform (free-living) larvae. These larvae may differentiate after a series of moults into free-living adults and repeat the cycle or metamorphose into the filariform larvae, which are infective to man.

(2) The parasitic cycle. Filariform larvae penetrate the skin, usually of the feet, and pass via the bloodstream to the lungs, where they break out into the alveolar spaces. After two additional moults, the adolescent larvae ascend the tracheobronchial tree to the glottis, are swallowed, and reach the upper small intestine, where the fertilized females burrow into the mucosa. The males are not tissue parasites and are voided in the feces. Deposition of eggs begins about 28 days after the initial infection. The thin-shelled eggs hatch rapidly within the intestinal wall or in the lumen, and the first-stage rhabditiform or noninfective larvae are passed in the feces. These larvae are 225 × 16 μm in size and have an elongated esophagus with a pyriform posterior bulb.

(3) Autoinfectious cycle. Sometimes development is accelerated; rhabditiform larvae moult and metamorphose into filariform larvae within the intestine. These infective forms, 550 μm in length, may penetrate the intestinal mucosa or the perianal skin and migrate to the small intestine via the lungs. This mechanism enables the infection to persist beyond the life-span of the adult females and may lead to the development of overwhelming infections.

Epidemiology

Transmission of *S. stercoralis* is facilitated by poor personal and public hygiene. Under optimal conditions of warmth, light, moisture, and oxygen, contamination of the soil with infected feces is followed by development of the free-living generation. When infective filariform larvae are formed, they may remain alive in the soil for several weeks. On contact with the skin or, rarely, with the buccal mucosa of man, the parasitic cycle is reinstituted. Contrary to most other helminth infections, the patient's worm burden is dependent not only on the intensity of exposure but also on the degree of autoinfection.

Disease Syndromes

Although millions of people throughout the world are infected with *S. stercoralis,* many individuals are asymptomatic or have only vague abdominal symptoms. Studies in institutions have shown that 15%–30% of individuals with proven strongyloidiasis are asymptomatic. Vague symptomatology in the remainder cannot be attributed wholly to strongyloidiasis because of the lack of comparison with uninfected controls.

(1) Cutaneous and pulmonary manifestations. These manifestations reflect the migration of the

parasite within the host. Penetration of the skin by filariform larvae usually produces little reaction, but repeated infection may result in the development of a pruritic, papular, erythematous rash. The frequency of pulmonary signs and symptoms is uncertain, but they are not strikingly common. Cough, shortness of breath, wheezing, and fever may develop as the larvae pass through the lungs. Transient pulmonary infiltrates have been observed on chest X-ray, and peripheral eosinophilia has been found.

(2) Intestinal manifestations. These manifestations begin with the invasion of the intestinal mucosa by the fertilized female worms and are the commonest mode of presentation of strongyloidiasis [1]. Abdominal pain occurs; it is often epigastric and burning in nature, is occasionally dull or crampy, and may be exacerbated by food. Diarrhea (with stools usually containing mucus) is common, sometimes alternating with constipation. Some patients complain of nausea and vomiting. These symptoms may be relatively acute in onset or may be chronic, with periodic attacks occurring for many years. Weight loss is common. Urticaria, observed in 5%–22% of cases, is usually generalized. Autoinfection by filariform larvae in the feces penetrating the perianal skin may cause larva currens; serpiginous wheals begin perianally and extend to the buttocks, abdomen, and thighs at rates of up to 10 cm per day [2]. Patients with chronic strongyloidiasis often present with an eosinophilia that may be the only sign of infection, although a normal eosinophil level in blood does not negate the diagnosis. In more severe infections, a malabsorption syndrome or protein-losing enteropathy may develop [3].

(3) Manifestations of hyperinfection. Autoinfection may lead to massive systemic strongyloidiasis, with severe, generalized, abdominal pain, distension, and shock [4]. A high fever frequently develops, and Gram-negative septicemia, which may lead to pneumonia or meningitis, is often found. Massive larval invasion of the lungs may result in cough, wheezing, and dyspnea; neurological signs may suggest cerebral involvement. Polymorphonuclear leukocytosis is common, but eosinophilia frequently does not develop.

The hyperinfection syndrome is being recognized increasingly in patients who are immunosuppressed either as a result of disease (lymphomas, leukemias, carcinomatosis, lepromatous leprosy, and kwashiorkor) or of therapy, particularly with corticosteroids [5, 6]. The syndrome may occur, however, in patients without an obvious predisposing cause.

Diagnosis

The process involved in the diagnosis and management of strongyloidiasis is illustrated in figure 1. Of crucial importance is the physician's suspicion of the presence of this helminth infection. The patient may present with abdominal pain, diarrhea, or eosinophilia; the sudden deterioration of an immunosuppressed patient should suggest the possibility of infection with *S. stercoralis.*

Once strongyloidiasis is suspected, a geographic history should be obtained. Although the distribution of this helminth infection is widespread, the diagnosis is more likely if the patient has been to the tropics or has lived in an area of known endemicity. A negative geographic history by no means rules out the diagnosis but renders it less likely.

Definitive diagnosis can be made only if larvae of *S. stercoralis* are found in the feces or duodenal fluid. The feces should be examined first. Larvae may sometimes be seen in simple smears, but it is better to employ a concentration technique. The zinc sulfate concentration method is the simplest.

A suspension is prepared by mixing 1 g or 1 ml of stool with 10 ml of warm tap water. The suspension is poured through a layer of damp gauze in a small funnel into a centrifuge tube, which is spun for 2 min at 1,000 *g*. The supernatant is decanted, and water (3 ml) is added. The sediment is resuspended by shaking, and the tube is filled with water and centrifuged as described above. This process is repeated until the supernatant becomes clear. The supernatant is then poured off, and a zinc sulfate solution (3 ml; 33 g/100 ml) is added. The sediment is resuspended, and more zinc sulfate solution is added until the tube is filled to about 1.5 cm from the top. The tube is then centrifuged at 2,000 *g* for 2 min. The surface film is transferred via a loop or pipette to a clean microscope slide, two drops of iodine solution (1% potassium iodide saturated with iodine) are mixed in, and the slide is examined at a magnification of ×100.

Examination of several stool samples may be necessary. Positive stools are found in about 70–80% of eventually diagnosed cases.

Negative stool findings necessitate sampling of duodenal contents either by intubation and aspiration or by the use of the Enterotest (Hedeco, Palo Alto, Calif.) [6]. This device consists of a gelatin capsule inside which is packed 140 cm of white nylon line. The capsule is swallowed by the patient, and the free end of the line is secured to the face and left in position for

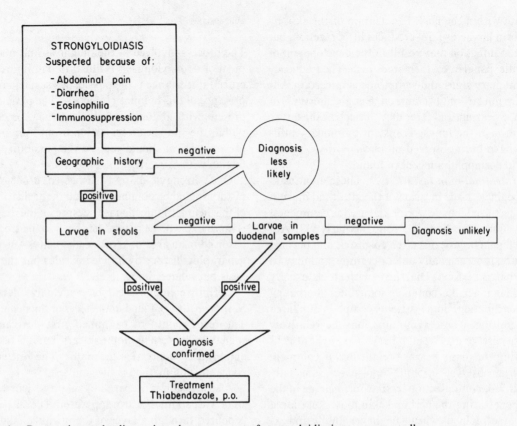

Figure 1. Progression to the diagnosis and management of strongyloidiasis; p.o. = perorally.

4 hr. In more than 95% of cases, the line extends to its full length and is carried into the duodenum by peristalsis. At this point the gelatin capsule has dissolved, and the line is removed by gentle traction. The distal portion of the nylon line, which is saturated with bile-stained mucus, is drawn through gloved fingers, and a few drops of duodenal contents are thereby expressed onto glass slides. The slides are examined at a magnification of ×100. In one study, *Strongyloides* larvae were found by this means in 51 of 56 persons thought to be infected [7]. If repeated fecal examinations and a satisfactory duodenal sample yield negative results, the patient is probably not infected. No effective immunological method is available for the diagnosis of strongyloidiasis.

Management

Since *Strongyloides* can multiply within the host, all infected patients should be treated, and the worms should be eradicated. Thiabendazole (Mintezol, Merck Sharpe and Dohme, West Point, Pa.) is given in a dose of 25 mg/kg twice daily for two days. Some patients may experience side effects such as anorexia, nausea, vomiting, dizziness, diarrhea, weariness, pruritis, and headache.

In the hyperinfection syndrome, it is essential that the diagnosis be made as rapidly as possible and that treatment be instituted early. Delay frequently results in death in spite of vigorous treatment. Patients with a past history of possible exposure to *Strongyloides* who are about to undergo immunosuppressive therapy should be examined for the parasite prior to the onset of treatment and followed carefully during therapy.

References

1. Jones, C. A. Clinical studies in human strongyloidiasis. I. Semeiology. Gastroenterology 16:743–756, 1950.
2. Smith, J. D., Goette, D. K., Odom, R. B. Larva currens: cutaneous strongyloidiasis. Arch. Dermatol. 112:1161–1163, 1976.
3. Milner, P. F., Irvine, R. A., Barton, C. J., Bras, G., Richards, R. Intestinal malabsorption in *Strongyloides stercoralis* infestation. Gut 6:574–581, 1965.

4. Bras, G., Richards, R. C., Irvine, R. A., Milner, P. F. A., Ragbeer, M. M. S. Infection with *Strongyloides stercoralis* in Jamaica. Lancet 2:1257–1260, 1964.

5. Rivera, E., Maldonado, N., Vēlez-Garcĭa, E., Grillo, A. J., Malaret, G. Hyperinfection syndrome with *Strongyloides stercoralis*. Ann. Intern. Med. 72:199–204, 1972.

6. Purtilo, D. T., Meyers, W. M., Connor, D. H. Fatal strongyloidiasis in immunosuppressed patients. Am. J. Med. 56:488–493, 1974.

7. Beal, C. B., Viens, P., Grant, R. G. L., Hughes, j. M. A new technique for sampling duodenal contents: demonstration of upper small bowel pathogens. Am. J. Trop. Med. Hyg. 19:349–352, 1970.

Tapeworms

Three major species of giant tapeworms, with mean lengths of 10–30 feet, may be found in the small intestines of man. The great size of these parasitic organisms has rendered them obvious since ancient times. All three tapeworms are transmitted by the ingestion of raw or undercooked flesh. *Taenia saginata* larvae are found in beef, those of *Taenia solium* in pork, and those of *Diphyllobothrium latum* in fish. The beef and fish tapeworms are distributed worldwide, with some transmission in the United States; the pork tapeworm is less widespread and is essentially an imported infection in the United States. Although these enormous intestinal helminths have been associated with abdominal and systemic disturbances, there is little definitive evidence for such symptomatology. Thus, the beef tapeworm appears to be essentially a benign, commensal organism. The larval stages of the pork tapeworm, however, can develop in man and spread throughout the body, including the brain; the lesions induced by these organisms are a major cause of epilepsy in some endemic areas. The fish tapeworm has a unique avidity for vitamin B_{12} and has been associated with the development of pernicious anemia in man. Recent drugs have rendered the treatment of the adult intestinal tapeworms a relatively sure and simple process.

Life Cycle

Infection of the definitive human host with a tapeworm follows the ingestion of raw, undercooked, or, perhaps, smoked flesh [1, 2]. In the case of *T. saginata* and *T. solium,* living larvae encysted in beef and pork (cysticerci, 5 × 10 mm in size), respectively, are digested out of the cysts, attach to the wall of the jejunum, and grow to maturity in several months. *D. latum* plerocercoids (worm-like larvae, 3 × 20 mm in size) from the tissue of fish pass down into the small intestine where they reach maturity in three to six weeks. The life span of all of these worms is measured in decades.

Tapeworms have a head (scolex) that is 1–2 mm in diameter; that of *T. solium* is crowned with hooklets, whereas that of *T. saginata* is bare, and both have four suckers. The *D. latum* scolex is almond-shaped with two suctorial grooves. From a small neck area that is 5–10 mm in length, a ribbon-like series of segments (proglottids) is constantly produced. Each proglottid develops into a self-contained hermaphroditic reproductive organism that produces large numbers of eggs from nutrients absorbed directly from the host. At maturity, the worms consist of 1,000 (*T. solium*), 2,000 (*T. saginata*), or 4,000 (*D. latum*) proglottids and vary in maximal length from 12 (*T. solium*) to 30 (*T. saginata* and *D. latum*) feet.

The mature proglottids of the two species of *Taenia,* which are 7 × 20 mm in size and contain 50,000 (*T. solium*)–80,000 (*T. saginata*) eggs, can be differentiated from one another, particularly by the number of lateral uterine branches. The proglottids break off from the terminal end of the worm; those of *T. solium* passively leave the body of the host, but those of *T. saginata* actively force their way out through the anus. Although *Taenia* eggs may be found in the stool, they are largely passed in the intact proglottids; and, in the case of *T. saginata,* an average of nine proglottids is passed per day [2]. The yellow-brown eggs of *Taenia* are approximately 35 μm in diameter and have a striated border with hooklets in the center; the eggs are identical in the two species of *Taenia.* The *D. latum* proglottids, which are 3 × 12 mm in size at maturity, produce and excrete within the intestinal lumen approximately one million yellow-brown operculate eggs daily (45 × 75 μm in size).

The *Taenia* eggs when deposited on the ground may be ingested by cattle (*T. saginata*) or pigs (*T. solium*) usually in small numbers, but occasionally an overwhelming infection may result from eating an entire proglottid. In the intestine the embryo is digested out of the eggs and is activated; these forms then penetrate the intestinal wall and spread throughout the tissues of the domestic animals, where they develop into mature infectious cysticerci within 10 weeks [3]. Whereas the eggs of *T. saginata* essentially do not develop into cysticerci in man, ingestion of the eggs of *T. solium* can lead to the development of cysticercosis; the sites of predilection are the subcutaneous tissues, brain, eyes, muscles, heart, liver, lungs, and peritoneum. *D. latum* eggs must enter fresh water to continue their development; the eggs first undergo a period of embryonation and then hatch into ciliated free-swimming coracidia. When the organisms are ingested by minute crustacea (copepods), they develop into elongated larvae. The copepods are then eaten by fish, and the larvae penetrate into the intestinal wall and lodge in the tissues where they grow and develop into the mature infective plerocercoid larvae.

Epidemiology

The two species of *Taenia* essentially have man as the only definitive host [1], whereas *D. latum* has been found in at least 22 species of fish-eating mammals. In the vast majority of infections, only one tapeworm is found in the human host. Distribution is largely related to the habit of eating raw, rare, or smoked flesh, and also to poor disposal of feces, which leads to infection of the respective intermediate hosts of the tapeworms. Thorough cooking destroys the cysticerci and plerocercoids; they are also killed by freezing.

T. saginata is found worldwide but is most prevalent in East Africa (>10%); a moderate prevalence of 0.5%–1.5% is seen in middle Europe, the Near East, and Central and South America. *T. saginata* is the most highly endemic, large tapeworm in the United States. Approximately 0.06% of federally inspected cattle are infected, and there is a minimal prevalence of 23 infected persons per 100,000 population [4]. The overall estimate is 200,000 cases in the United States today. Infection is more common among the affluent than the poor. *T. solium* is reportedly much less prevalent globally and is seen most frequently in South Africa, Mexico, India, the Slavic countries of Europe, northern China, Brazil, and Chile. This parasite is not endemic in the United States and is seen only rarely (e.g., one of 81 cases of *Taenia* infection recently reported in this country). *D. latum* is particularly common in the northern lake country of Scandinavia (Finland has the highest prevalence, 20–60%), northern Europe, Siberia, northern China, Canada, Argentina, and Chile. In the United States *D. latum* can be found in the lake regions of Wisconsin, Minnesota, and Michigan, and cases have been reported in New York City and Florida [4]. *D. latum* is also quite commonly seen in Alaskan Eskimos.

Disease Syndromes

In a complete zoological overview of the pathogenesis of adult cestodes, it was stated that these organisms "have little effect on the host and are rarely pathogenic" [1]. Infection with many worms can result in disease, but a human host almost always harbors only one tapeworm. In a massive review of the literature on *T. saginata* infections, it was noted that the passage of motile proglottids through the anus is noticed by 98% of patients [2]. The next most frequent symptom was abdominal pain (36%) which was followed by a long list of others. None of these clinical studies, however, appears to have been done with appropriate uninfected control groups.

In a questionnaire-type investigation of symptoms of carriers of *D. latum* without anemia, a large group of uninfected controls was included [5]. The incidence of abdominal pain in carriers (45%) was not significantly different from that in controls (4). Significant differences in the following symptoms were noted in carriers vs. controls: "not perfectly healthy," 59% vs. 44%; "craving for salt," 62% vs. 42%; "diarrhea," 22% vs. 10%; "fatigue and weakness," 66% vs. 50%; "dizziness," 53% vs. 39%; and "numbness of extremities," 49% vs. 37%. With the exception of diarrhea, abdominal signs and symptoms were essentially absent. Concerning general well-being, although many of the differences were statistically significant, it is difficult to come to any strong conclusions because of the high level of positive findings in the controls. Although statements such as "there is sometimes a variable eosinophilia" are often made, eosinophilia has not been clearly demonstrated in infections with these organisms, which dwell within the lumen of the intestines. A specific study of this problem revealed that eosinophilia does not occur in *D. latum* infections [1].

According to folklore, tapeworms utilize significant amounts of the nutriment available to the definitive hosts. However, calculations made with *T. saginata* revealed that, even though these organisms produce an average of nine proglottids daily and thus manufacture the equivalent of 500 million eggs per year, the total amount of worm produced per year is less than two pounds [1]. With *D. latum,* however, the absorption by the worm of a specific dietary substance does lead to disease. *D. latum* has a great affinity for vitamin B_{12} (e.g., 50 times that of *T. saginata* [1]), and the higher the worm is located in the small intestine, the greater the absorption of vitamin B_{12}. In Finland, where *D. latum* infection is extremely common, it has been estimated that 0.1% of the infected population develop pernicious anemia; in some areas the estimate is up to 2%. Megaloblastic bone marrow is seen, and subacute degeneration of the spinal cord has been reported.

Although invasion of the tissues of man with the larval forms of *T. saginata* is exceedingly rare, it does occur quite frequently with *T. solium* [3]. As far as is known, cysticercosis can develop only by the direct ingestion of embryonated eggs; in this process the eggs must pass through the stomach in order to hatch. Although it has often been suggested that "internal autoinfection" by reverse peristalsis occurs, there is no recorded proof of this phenomenon [3]. As in the pig, the larval form of *T. solium* is found throughout the tissues of the human body, including the brain. The larvae in the cortical tissue are walled off by a capsule of sclerosed neuroglia and do not usually provoke symptoms until degeneration of the cysticercus begins, which usually takes several years. An inflammatory reaction occurs upon degeneration of the cysticercus, and one of the major symptoms is epilepsy, the most frequent of the neurological complications of cysticercosis. Most of the seizures are generalized, although some are focal. Occasionally, cysticerci can block the ventricular system of the brain resulting in raised intracranial pressure. Organisms within the eye can cause significant damage, as can those within the cardiac musculature. Eosinophilia is not a common concomitant of cysticercosis.

Diagnosis

As can be seen in figure 1, it is likely that most patients with tapeworm will consult a physician because they have felt the motile proglottids of *T. saginata* pass through the anus or have noted taenia proglottids or large portions of any of the three cestodes in the feces. The presence of pernicious anemia suggests the possibility of *D. latum* infection. Whether infections with these organisms cause abdominal or systemic symptomatology remains questionable except under unusual conditions such as when there are multiple parasites.

The geographic history of the patient is helpful in diagnosis. Although *T. saginata* can occur virtually anywhere, it is far more prevalent in certain areas, such as East Africa. *D. latum* is also widespread and is particularly common in Finland. In the United States, it is usually found in the northern lake regions and in Alaska. *T. solium* has a more specific geo-

graphic distribution and is not endemic in the United States.

A history of the frequent ingestion of raw or undercooked flesh is a strong positive clue, but infection may also occur in those who eat rare meat only occasionally or even in those who do so inadvertently.

Fecal examination for eggs of *Taenia* species requires some form of concentration of the stool. With a thick smear system such as the Kato, three separate fecal examinations should result in the diagnosis of as many as 97% of cases [2]. A 20-mg sample of feces that has been pressed through 105-mesh stainless steel bolting cloth (W. S. Tyler, Cleveland, Ohio) is placed on a glass slide and covered with a cellophane coverslip (no. 124 PD, Film Department, E. I. DuPont de Nemours, Wilmington, Del.) impregnated with 50% glycerine. The slides are inverted, pressed onto a bed of filter paper, turned face up, and left for a period of 15 minutes, during which time the fecal matter clears and the eggs can be easily seen. It is also worthwhile to examine the perianal skin with the scotch-tape method. The eggs of the two species of *Taenia* cannot be differentiated. The large and characteristic eggs of *D. latum,* however, are quite simple to detect in the feces since they are released in the intestinal tract in very large numbers.

Although the mature proglottids of the two *Taenia* species are different, particularly in the number of uterine branches, their definitive identification usually requires the use of special fixation and staining procedures. Proglottids of *D. latum* are quite different from those of the two *Taenia* species and are easily identified. Since the treatment of all of the tapeworms is now the same, identification of the specific species of *Taenia* is not necessary.

With respect to cysticercosis, epilepsy or other neurological syndromes confined to the central nervous system in someone from a region endemic for *T. solium* infection suggests the possibility of the diagnosis. A history of infection with tapeworm should be sought and the patient should be examined for such infection, even though it is found in less than one-third of the cases. X rays of the soft tissues may reveal the presence of calcified cysticerci although the organisms in the brain rarely calcify. Serologic testing is also of value, and a hemagglutination test has been shown to yield 85% positivity in patients with cysticercosis that has been proven by radiology or biopsy [6]. In a random population the incidence of false positive results was 5%, and in patients known to be carriers of pork tapeworm, 17% [6].

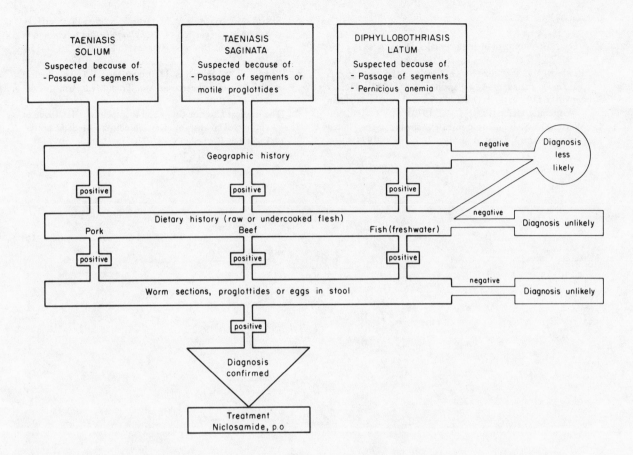

Figure 1. The progression to the diagnosis and treatment of tapeworms; p.o. = perorally.

Management

For all three tapeworm infections, niclosamide (Yomesan®) is the treatment of choice [7]. This drug can be obtained from the Parasitic Drug Service of the Center for Disease Control, Atlanta, Georgia. Four tablets (2 g) are chewed thoroughly in a single dose after a light meal (88% of cases are cured on first treatment). Failure of therapy can be followed by a second dose of niclosamide. The patient should be reassured of the essential harmlessness of the intestinal phase of these organisms. Surgery is rarely indicated in cerebral cysticercosis, and treatment should be largely palliative and directed toward the control of epilepsy.

Dwarf Tapeworm

The dwarf tapeworm, *Hymenolepis nana,* is found most commonly in children in warm climates. In the United States, it is usually found in the southeast, with prevalences ranging from 0.3% in Florida to 2.9% in Tennessee [4]. The average length of this organism is 2 cm, and it consists of as many as 200 proglottids. The gravid segments contain 80–180 eggs which are released within the intestines. Infection is usually by person-to-person transmission via ingestion of eggs, but autoinfection may also occur. The life cycle of *H. nana* is completed with a stage of development within the intestinal villus, and the adult worms reside in the lumen of the ileum.

The clinical and public health importance of *H. nana* infection is uncertain, although children with heavy worm burdens have been reported to have intestinal and systemic symptoms. Diagnosis is made by fecal examination, which reveals the 40- $\times$ 50-μm eggs that contain embryos with characteristic hooklets. Niclosamide is again the drug of choice, and treatment is administered for five days in a dose of 2 g per day for adults [7] and 40 mg/kg daily for children.

References

1. Rees, G. Pathogenesis of adult cestodes. Helm. Abs. 36:1–23, 1967.
2. Pawlowski, Z., Schultz, M. G. Taeniasis and cysticercosis (*Taenia saginata*). Adv. Parasitol. 10:269–343, 1972.
3. Smyth, J. D., Heath, D. D. Pathogenesis of larval cestodes in mammals. Helm. Abs. 39:1–22, 1970.
4. Warren, K. S. Helminthic diseases endemic in the United States. Am. J. Trop. Med. Hyg. 23:723–730, 1974.
5. Saarni, M., Nybergy, W., Gräsbeck, R., von Bonsdorff, B. Symptoms in carriers of *Diphyllobothrium latum* and in non-infected controls. Acta Med. Scand. 173:147–154, 1963.
6. Proctor, E. M., Powell, S. J., Elsdon-Dew, R. The serological diagnosis of cysticercosis. Ann. Trop. Med. Parasitol. 60: 146–151, 1966.
7. The medical letter on drugs and therapeutics. Handbook of antimicrobial therapy. Revised edition. Medical Letter, Inc., New Rochelle, N.Y., 1976, pp. 60–61.

Trichinosis

Trichinosis, an infection with the nematode *Trichinella spiralis,* may occur after the ingestion of the undercooked flesh of any carnivore, but it is usually associated with pork. Most infections are asymptomatic but heavy exposure, often occurring in limited epidemics, results in clinical disease characterized by periorbital edema, myositis, and fever. Treatment is unsatisfactory and severe infections may be fatal.

T. spiralis has a worldwide distribution with the exceptions of Australia and many of the Pacific islands. It is found throughout the United States but is most prevalent in the northeast and on the west coast. Although the prevalence of trichinosis is declining, it remains one of the most important helminthic infections in the United States because of its potential severity. In a nationwide autopsy survey in 1941, 16% of cadavers were positive for trichinellae, but by 1968 the number of infected cadavers had fallen to 4% [1]. Similarly, the number of reported cases has declined from 500 in 1948 to around 100 in recent years; 20 deaths have been reported during the last 10 years.

Life Cycle

When viable larvae of *T. spiralis* are ingested in raw or inadequately cooked meat, the organisms are freed from the cyst walls by acid-pepsin digestion and pass into the small intestine, where they attach to the villi. After moulting, the trichinellae develop into adult worms; males are $1,500 \times 50$ μm and females $3,500 \times 60$ μm in size. Each fertilized female worm releases approximately 500 larvae (100×5 μm in size) during a period of two weeks, after which the adult worms are eliminated from the gut. The larvae, which seed the skeletal muscles by way of the lymphatics and blood vessels, burrow into individual muscle fibers; during a period of three weeks the larvae increase 10 times in length and become coiled, resistant to acid-pepsin digestion, and capable of infecting a new host. A cyst wall of muscle origin that develops around the larvae may calcify during the next few months or years. Encysted larvae may remain viable for several years, and when they are ingested by other animals the cycle of trichinosis continues.

Epidemiology

Trichinosis is essentially a zoonosis; man is an incidental host. The organism is widely spread in nature among a large number of carnivorous animals, including rats, pigs, bears, cats, dogs, foxes, opossums, and raccoons. In a survey in Iowa, up to 5% of such animals were found to be infected [2]. Pigs become infected chiefly from eating uncooked scraps of pig meat or occasionally wild animals, particularly rats. The vast majority of swine in the United States are grain-fed, and only 0.1% are infected with trichinellae. While the remainder (1.5%) are garbage-fed, legislation introduced in the middle 1950s forbidding the feeding of uncooked garbage has reduced *T. spiralis* infection in pigs from 10% to 0.5%.

Man usually contracts the infection by eating inadequately processed pork; for example, in 1971 pork products were incriminated as the source of infection in 71% of cases reported to the Center for Disease Control. Beef products such as hamburger may become adulterated with pork through the use of a common meat grinder or the intentional mixing of meats. Bear meat is an occasional cause of epidemics of human trichinosis [3]. Asymptomatic infection probably results from light exposure either as a result of eating inadequately cooked meat in which most but not all of the cysts are destroyed or as a result of dilution of infectious meat in large packing houses. Preexisting immunity may also reduce the infectivity of an inoculum of larvae. Strains of *T. spiralis* with various degrees of infectivity have also been reported. Epidemics occur when families or small communities consume trichinous meat from a common source.

Smoking, salting, and drying do not destroy infective larvae. Meat can be sterilized by adequate freezing; for example, a cut six inches thick is safe after storing at -15 C (the temperature of the average home freezer) for 20 days, but the most effective method is proper cooking. The thermal death point of trichinellae is 55 C, so that meat should be cooked until there is no trace of pink fluid or flesh.

Disease Syndromes

The vast majority of infections in man are subclinical; the development of symptoms depends mainly on the size of the inoculum of viable larvae. The minimal number of larvae required to produce symptoms is said to be about 100, while a fatal dose is of the order of 300,000. Most of the infected subjects in the 1968 national autopsy survey [1] had low worm burdens: 38% had less than one larva, and 52% had one to 10 larvae per g of muscle; 9% had 10–100 larvae, and only 1% had more than 100 larvae per g of muscle. The clinical features in heavily infected individuals reflect the intestinal and muscle stages in the life cycle of the parasite.

(1) Intestinal manifestations. Symptoms attributable to the adult worms in the intestines are much less common than those associated with invasion of muscle by the larvae, but when they occur they are found during the first week after infection. Diarrhea is seen in about 40% of patients in epidemics; the stools are of variable consistency and are sometimes blood-stained. Abdominal discomfort afflicts 20% and vomiting develops in 10% of cases. Patients with extremely heavy worm burdens may die from fulminant enteritis during this phase of the infection.

(2) Eye and muscle manifestations. Symptoms due to invasion of the muscles by larvae usually appear during the second week after infection, often around the 10th day. Fever is found in 90% of symptomatic patients, although it is variable in intensity and duration. Periorbital edema is usually the first physical sign, occurring in 80% of cases, and in severe infections may spread to other parts of the face; subconjunctival hemorrhages and chemosis also may be seen. Myalgia, often associated with muscle swelling and weakness, is seen in 80% of patients. It frequently begins in the extraocular muscles and then develops in the masseters, neck muscles, tongue, flexor muscles of the extremities, and lumbar muscles. Half of the patients complain of headache, and many have cough, shortness of breath, hoarseness, and dysphagia. A rash, often macular in nature, is seen in about 10% of subjects. Occasionally there are neurological or urological symptoms.

In most patients the symptoms reach a peak at two to three weeks of infection. Thereafter the fever abates and muscle symptoms slowly subside, but malaise and weakness may persist for weeks. Fatalities have been reported in about 2% of symptomatic patients;

the usual cause of death is a nonspecific interstitial myocarditis (larvae do not encyst in cardiac muscle), but deaths are occasionally related to encephalitis or pneumonia.

Diagnosis

The process involved in the diagnosis of trichinosis is illustrated in the accompanying algorithm (figure 1). The infection may be suspected in a patient who presents with periorbital edema, myositis, and fever. At times, an otherwise asymptomatic patient may have eosinophilia. An epidemiological and dietary history should be taken, and if others who have eaten the same meat have similar symptoms the likelihood of the diagnosis is greatly increased. The infection is unlikely if intensive questioning fails to elicit any history of eating the inadequately cooked meat of pigs or other carnivores (particularly bears), but it must be remembered that some commercial beef products have pork additives.

The peripheral blood should then be examined for eosinophilia, which usually begins on about the 10th day after infection, is found in 90% of patients with clinical trichinosis, and sometimes reaches very high levels. If there is no eosinophilia, the diagnosis is less likely. Determinations of enzymes in serum may be useful indicators of muscle involvement. The level of creatine phosphokinase is elevated in half of the patients and the level of lactic dehydrogenase in somewhat more.

The skin test for *Trichinella* does not differentiate between past and recent infection, but serological tests (particularly bentonite flocculation) may be useful in establishment of the diagnosis. The advantage of this test is that titers of antibody fall to low levels within two years after infection, and thus the diagnosis of reinfection is facilitated. Unfortunately, levels of antibody are not detectable until three weeks after infection or longer, although 99% of subjects will eventually become positive; a titer of 1:5 or a fourfold rise in titer is considered to be of diagnostic significance [4]. Serum (1 ml) may be sent at ambient temperature to the Center for Disease Control (Atlanta, Ga.) for testing.

If a patient has a positive epidemiological and dietary history, eosinophilia, and positive serological results, then the diagnosis is probable, and it is unnecessary to proceed to muscle biopsy. Doubt may be resolved by taking a biopsy specimen from a tender

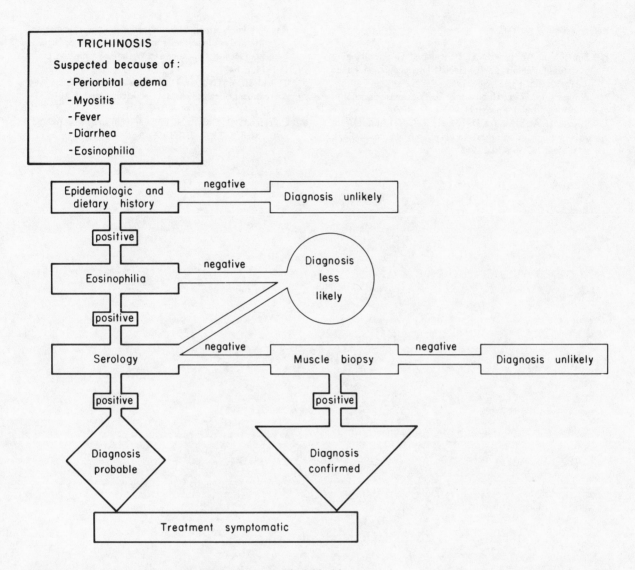

Figure 1. The progression to a definitive diagnosis of trichinosis.

swollen muscle at least three weeks after the presumed onset of infection; by this means the chances of obtaining a positive result are increased because of increased numbers of larvae, their greater size, and large inflammatory reactions. In epidemics, the number of positive biopsy specimens has varied between 25% and 100% but is usually closer to the higher figure. If the biopsy specimen is positive, the diagnosis is confirmed.

Management

The treatment of trichinosis is unsatisfactory [5, 6]. Thiabendazole (Mintezole,® Merck, Sharpe and

Dohme, West Point, Pa.) may eliminate intestinal worms if given within one day of ingestion of larvae. In rare instances, when there is a localized epidemic and a patient is known to have ingested trichinous meat recently, the drug should be administered in a dose of 25 mg/kg twice daily for one week. Usually, however, the diagnosis is not made until two weeks or more after infection. At this time, thiabendazole has no effect on the numbers of larvae in muscle, nor does it significantly alter the course of the disease. The mainstay of therapy is the administration of antiinflammatory analgesic agents such as salicylates. Critically ill patients may be treated with corticosteroids, but the evidence for benefit is equivocal.

References

1. Zimmerman, W. J., Steele, J. H., Kagan, I. G. The changing status of trichiniasis in the United States population. Public Health Rep. 83:957–966, 1968.
2. Zimmerman, W. J., Hubbard, E. D. Trichiniasis in wildlife of Iowa. Am. J. Epidemiol. 90:84–92, 1969.
3. Roselle, H. A., Schwartz, D. T., Geer, F. G. Trichinosis from New England bear meat: report of an epidemic. N. Engl. J. Med. 272:304–305, 1965.
4. Kagan, I. G., Norman, L. Serodiagnosis of parasitic disease. *In* Manual of clinical microbiology. 2nd ed. U.S. Department of Health, Education and Welfare, Washington, D.C., 1974, p. 645.
5. Thibadeau, Y., Gagnon, J. Trichinosis: thiabendazole in the treatment of eleven cases. Can. Med. Assoc. J. 101:533–536, 1965.
6. Corridan, J. P., Gray, J. J. Trichinosis in southwest Ireland. Br. Med. J. 2:727–730, 1969.

Trichuriasis

Trichuriasis, or whipworm, is among the most prevalent of all the helminthic parasites of mankind; a conservative estimate is that more than half a billion individuals are infected [1]. A recent survey of the literature suggested that there are 2.2 million individuals with trichuriasis in the continental United States, mainly in the rural southeast. A large-scale study in Puerto Rico revealed a 75% infection rate in six-year-old children. *Trichuris trichiura* has an exceedingly simple life cycle, in which ingested eggs hatch in the small bowel and the larvae pass directly down into their final habitat in the colon. The head of the worm is embedded in the mucosa, from which it appears to take up minute amounts of blood. Most individuals with trichuriasis have relatively light infections of no clinical significance. Heavy infections, which occur mainly in young children, may result in some disease manifestations. Whereas treatment in the past has been inadequate, an effective nontoxic drug has recently been developed.

Life Cycle

Adult *T. trichiura* (males, 38 mm in length; females, 43 mm) have a relatively long, attenuated, whip-like anterior portion and a shorter, thicker, handle-like posterior end [1]. The normal habitat of the worms is the cecum and ascending colon, but in heavy infections they may be found throughout the entire large bowel. The anterior tip of the parasite is inserted into the intestinal tissues, from which the organism sucks blood in minute quantities. The mean life-span of *Trichuris* is several years; during this period the female worms daily produce approximately 7,500 characteristic, barrel-shaped eggs with transparent polar plugs ($50 \times 20 \mu m$). After excretion in the feces, the eggs embryonate under optimal conditions of moisture and shade in two to four weeks. After ingestion of embryonated eggs by the human host, the larval worms hatch in the small intestine, where they remain for several days among the intestinal villi. The adolescent worms then slowly pass down into the cecal area, where they develop into mature, egg-producing adults in 30–90 days.

Epidemiology

While man is the principal host of *T. trichiura,* the presence of this parasite has also been recorded in monkeys, lemurs, and hogs [1]. Trichuriasis is most common in rural areas where there is a lack of sanitation. Shade and moisture are the optimal conditions for the development of the eggs, which are readily destroyed by sunlight and desiccation. Thus, while *Trichuris* and *Ascaris* are both spread widely throughout the tropics, the latter is more common in dry and the former in moist climates. The intensity of *Trichuris* infection is greatest in children, particularly in those two to three years of age who most frequently come into contact with soil. The infection is also spread by fecally contaminated fruits and vegetables and can be transferred to foodstuffs by flies.

Disease Syndromes

Although trichuriasis is exceedingly prevalent worldwide, disease appears to occur only in a very small proportion of those infected and to be related to the worm burden. Since the most intense infections are usually in children, it is not surprising that almost all of the disease attributed to this parasite is seen in the young. These children often suffer from multiple parasitic infections and malnutrition, and it has been difficult to determine the role of *T. trichiura* in the disease syndromes.

The direct contact of parasite and host at the site where the head of the helminth is embedded in the intestinal mucosa is associated with no pathological reaction other than slight cytolysis without definite inflammatory reaction [2]. In one careful study in which radioactive chromium-tagged red blood cells were used, uptake of blood averaging 0.005 ml per worm per day was demonstrated [3]. This uptake is, respectively, eight and 40 times less than that noted for the hookworms *Necator* and *Ancylostoma*. The authors of this study claim that some degree of anemia may occur in young children with exceedingly heavy infections ($\geqslant$800 worms). In a more recent

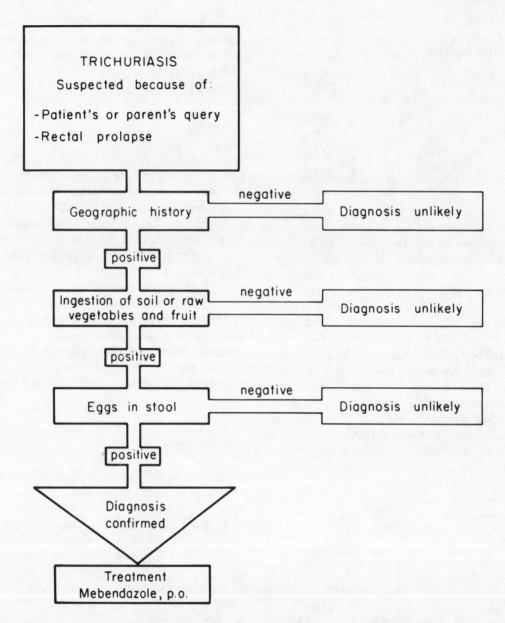

Figure 1.   The progression to the diagnosis and management of trichuriasis; p.o. = perorally.

study, however, in which similar methodology was used, it was reported that, in otherwise healthy children with heavy trichuris infections (mean, 406 worms), blood loss was within the accepted normal range for persons without parasitic infection. Since the vast majority of worm burdens are well below the above levels, trichuriasis can be considered to be only a rare cause of anemia.

Studies of eosinophilia in schoolchildren in whom the intensity of trichuris infection was determined and in an uninfected control group led to the statement

that "it seems probable that no eosinophilia is elicited by chronic whipworm infection" [4].

A plethora of abdominal signs and symptoms has been reported in trichuriasis, including pain and bloody diarrhea. Most investigations into the disease, however, have been performed in patients who entered the hospital because of abdominal complaints. In many cases, there have been multiple intestinal helminthic infections and associated malnutrition. One investigator found that diarrhea and dysentery occurred most frequently in the children with the heaviest egg counts, but this group also had an inordinately high prevalence of amebiasis [5]. Careful autopsies of two children with massive infections revealed no lesions attributable to the parasites; both patients had concomitant *Entamoeba histolytica* infections [2]. Rectal prolapse has been repeatedly reported in young children with heavy trichuris infections [5].

In summary, trichuriasis appears to be an essentially nonpathogenic helminthic infection. Massively infected young children may suffer from mild anemia, bloody diarrhea (although this may be due largely to amebiasis), and/or rectal prolapse.

Diagnosis

The progression to a diagnosis of trichuriasis is shown in figure 1. As is mentioned above, a significant degree of infection accompanied by disease manifestations is most likely in young children from tropical and semitropical areas. In the United States the majority of such patients will come from the southeastern states or Puerto Rico. A positive geographic history should be followed by careful questioning about contact of young children with soil and ingestion of raw, nonpeelable vegetables and fruits by those of all ages. This interview is followed by stool examination as described below.

Since the eggs of *Trichuris* are so characteristic in appearance and since the level of egg output is so high (about 200 eggs/g of feces per worm pair), the infection can be readily diagnosed by simple fecal smear. For the direct smear, a drop of saline is placed on a microscope slide, a small portion of feces is emulsified in the solution, and a coverslip is placed on top of it. The density of the preparation should be such that fine print can be read through the smear [6]. These preparations usually contain between 1.0 and 1.5 mg of feces; for estimation of the number of eggs per g of feces, the egg count is usually multiplied by 750. This method should reliably detect as few as five worm pairs. If the findings are negative, it is not

necessary to use more sensitive methods to detect the eggs, as it has been suggested that symptomatology appears only in infections with > 30,000 eggs/g of feces or in those with > 150 worm pairs.

Management

First, it is important to point out that it is unnecessary to treat patients with low egg counts. This assertion was especially valid in the past when the only drugs available for the treatment of trichuriasis were both ineffective and toxic. The recent introduction of the oral drug mebendazole (Vermox,® Ortho Pharmaceutical Corp., Raritan, N.J.), however, has totally changed the situation. This drug is poorly absorbed from the gastrointestinal tract, and essentially no side effects follow its use. The recommended dose of 100 mg twice a day for three days, regardless of body weight, gives a cure rate of 70%–96% and a reduction in egg output of 90%–99% [7]. Even though cure may not be achieved, the marked reduction in worm burden renders retreatment unnecessary.

References

1. Belding, D. L. Textbook of parasitology. 3rd ed. Appleton-Century-Crofts, New York, 1965, p. 397–402.
2. Hartz, P. H. Histopathology of the colon in massive trichocephaliasis in children. Doc. Med. Geog. Trop. 5:303–313, 1953.
3. Layrisse, M., Aparcedo, L., Martinez-Torres, C., Roche, M. Blood loss due to infection with *Trichuris trichiura*. Am. J. Trop. Med. Hyg. 16:613–619, 1967.
4. Otto, G. F. Blood studies on *Trichuris*-infested and worm-free children in Louisiana. Am. J. Trop. Med. 15:693–704, 1935.
5. Jung, R. C., Beaver, P. C. Clinical observations on *Trichocephalus trichiurus* (whipworm) infestation in children. Pediatrics 8:548–557, 1951.
6. Melvin, D. M., Brooke, M. M. Laboratory procedures for the diagnosis of intestinal parasites. U.S. Department of Health, Education, and Welfare (publication no. [CDC] 75-8282), Atlanta, 1974, p. 37, 38, 165.
7. Mebendazole—a new anthelmintic. Med. Lett. Drugs Ther. 17:37–38, 1975.

Contributors

Butler, T., M.D.   Assistant Professor of Medicine, Division of Geographic Medicine, Department of Medicine, Case Western Reserve University; Assistant Physician, University Hospitals of Cleveland.

Carpenter, C. C. J., M.D.   John H. Hord Chairman and Director, Department of Medicine; Adjunct Member, Division of Geographic Medicine; Case Western Reserve University and University Hospitals of Cleveland.

Daniel, T. M., M.D.   Professor of Medicine, Division of Pulmonary Diseases; Adjunct Member, Division of Geographic Medicine; Department of Medicine, Case Western Reserve University; Physician, University Hospitals of Cleveland.

Grove, D. I., M.D.   Assistant Professor of Medicine, Division of Geographic Medicine, Department of Medicine, Case Western Reserve University; Assistant Physician, University Hospitals of Cleveland.

Lozoff, B., M.D.   Assistant Professor of Medicine and Pediatrics; Division of Geographic Medicine, Department of Medicine and Department of Pediatrics, Case Western Reserve University; Assistant Physician, University Hospitals of Cleveland.

Mahmoud, A. A. F., M.D., Ph.D.   Associate Professor of Medicine, Director, Division of Geographic Medicine, Department of Medicine, Case Western Reserve University; Associate Physician, University Hospitals of Cleveland.

Robbins, F. C., M.D.   Dean of the School of Medicine; Professor of Pediatrics and of Community Health; Adjunct Member, Division of Geographic Medicine, Department of Medicine, Case Western Reserve University.

Stevens, D. P., M.D.   Assistant Professor of Medicine, Divisions of Gastroenterology and Geographic Medicine, Department of Medicine, Case Western Reserve University; Assistant Physician, University Hospitals of Cleveland.

Warren, K. S., M.D.   Director for Health Sciences, The Rockefeller Foundation. Formerly, Professor of Medicine; Director, Division of Geographic Medicine, Department of Medicine; Professor of Library Science, Case Western Reserve University; Associate Physician, University Hospitals of Cleveland.

Index